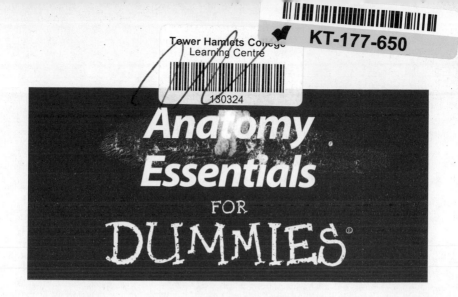

Anatomy Essentials

FOR

DUMMIES®

TOWER HAMLETS COLLEGE
POPLAR HIGH STREET
LONDON
E14 0AF

by Maggie Norris and
Donna Rae Siegfried
with Medhane Cumbay

WILEY

John Wiley & Sons, Inc.

Anatomy Essentials For Dummies®

Published by
John Wiley & Sons, Inc.
111 River St.
Hoboken, NJ 07030-5774
www.wiley.com

Copyright © 2012 by John Wiley & Sons, Inc., Hoboken, New Jersey

Published simultaneously in Canada

For general information on our other products and services, please contact our Customer Care Department within the U.S. at 877-762-2974, outside the U.S. at 317-572-3993, or fax 317-572-4002.

For technical support, please visit www.wiley.com/techsupport.

Wiley publishes in a variety of print and electronic formats and by print-on-demand. Some material included with standard print versions of this book may not be included in e-books or in print-on-demand. If this book refers to media such as a CD or DVD that is not included in the version you purchased, you may download this material at http://booksupport.wiley.com. For more information about Wiley products, visit www.wiley.com.

Library of Congress Control Number: 2012936855

ISBN 978-1-118-18421-9 (pbk); ISBN 978-1-118-22748-0 (ebk); ISBN 978-1-118-24039-7 (ebk); ISBN 978-1-118-26512-3 (ebk)

Manufactured in the United States of America

10 9 8 7 6 5 4 3 2 1

WILEY

About the Authors

Maggie Norris is a freelance science writer living in the San Francisco Bay area. As Fine Print Publication Services LLB, Maggie offers contract medical and technical writing services to clients in the pharmaceutical, biotech, and medical technology industries; patient care institutions; and research institutions.

Donna Rae Siegfried has written about pharmaceutical and medical topics for 15 years in publications, including *Prevention, Runner's World, Men's Health,* and *Organic Gardening.* She has taught anatomy and physiology at the college level. She is also the co-author of *Biology For Dummies,* 2nd Edition (Wiley).

Publisher's Acknowledgments

We're proud of this book; please send us your comments at http://dummies.custhelp.com. For other comments, please contact our Customer Care Department within the U.S. at 877-762-2974, outside the U.S. at 317-572-3993, or fax 317-572-4002.

Some of the people who helped bring this book to market include the following:

Acquisitions, Editorial, and Vertical Websites

Project Editor: Jennifer Tebbe

Acquisitions Editor: Stacy Kennedy

Copy Editors: Jennette ElNaggar, Jessica Smith

Assistant Editor: David Lutton

Editorial Program Coordinator: Joe Niesen

Technical Editors: Scott Houser, Sara Newton

Editorial Manager: Christine Meloy Beck

Editorial Assistants: Rachelle S. Amick, Alexa Koschier

Art Coordinator: Alicia B. South

Cartoons: Rich Tennant (www.the5thwave.com)

Composition Services

Project Coordinator: Patrick Redmond

Layout and Graphics: Corrie Niehaus, Laura Westhuis, Erin Zeltner

Proofreaders: Bryan Coyle, John Greenough

Indexer: Potomac Indexing, LLC

Illustrator: Kathryn Born

Publishing and Editorial for Consumer Dummies

Kathleen Nebenhaus, Vice President and Executive Publisher

Kristin Ferguson-Wagstaffe, Product Development Director

Ensley Eikenburg, Associate Publisher, Travel

Kelly Regan, Editorial Director, Travel

Publishing for Technology Dummies

Andy Cummings, Vice President and Publisher

Composition Services

Debbie Stailey, Director of Composition Services

Contents at a Glance

Table of Contents

Introduction

C ongratulations on your decision to study human anatomy and physiology. The knowledge you gain from your study is of value in many aspects of your life.

A little background in anatomy and physiology should be considered a valuable part of anyone's education. Health and medical matters are part of world events and people's daily lives. Basic knowledge of anatomy and physiology gets you started when trying to make sense of the news about epidemics, novel drugs and medical devices, and purported environmental hazards, to name just a few examples. Everyone has a problem with some aspect of his or her anatomy and physiology at some point, and this knowledge can help you be a better parent, spouse, caregiver, neighbor, friend, or colleague.

Knowledge of anatomy and physiology may also benefit your own health. Sometimes, comprehension of a particular fact or concept can help drive a good decision about long-term health matters, such as the demonstrated benefits of exercise, or it may help you take appropriate action in the context of a specific medical problem, such as an infection, a cut, or a muscle strain. You may understand your doctors' instructions better during a course of treatment, which may give you a better medical outcome.

About This Book

Anatomy Essentials For Dummies guides you on a quick walk-through of human anatomy and physiology. It doesn't have the same degree of technical detail as a textbook. It contains relatively little in the way of lists of important anatomical structures, for instance. We expect that most readers are using this book as a complementary resource for course work in anatomy and physiology at the high-school or college level. Therefore, the goals of this book are to be informal but not unscientific, brief but not sketchy, and information-rich but accessible to readers at many levels.

Conventions Used in This Book

We use the following conventions throughout the text to make the presentation of information consistent and easy to understand:

- ✔ New terms appear in *italic* and are closely followed by an easy-to-understand definition.
- ✔ **Bold** is used to highlight keywords in bulleted lists.

If you're using this book as a supplement to an assigned textbook, note that your course materials may name structures and physiological substances using a different nomenclature (naming system) than the one we use in this book.

Foolish Assumptions

We're guessing that you fall into one of these categories:

- ✔ **Formal student:** You're a high-school or college student enrolled in a basic anatomy and physiology course for credit. You need to pass an exam or otherwise demonstrate understanding and retention of data, terminology, and concepts in human anatomy and physiology.
- ✔ **Informal student:** You're not enrolled in a credit course, but gaining some background in human anatomy and physiology is important to you for personal or professional reasons.
- ✔ **Casual reader:** Here you are with a book on your hands and a little time to spend reading it. And it's all about you!

Icons Used in This Book

The little round pictures that you see in the margins throughout this book are icons that alert you to different kinds of valuable information.

This icon serves to highlight information we think you should permanently store in your mental anatomy and physiology file.

The bull's-eye symbol lets you know what you can do to improve your understanding of an anatomical structure.

Where to Go from Here

If you're currently enrolled in (or planning to enroll in) a formal course in human anatomy and physiology, you may get the most benefit by becoming familiar with this book a week or two before your course begins. Peruse the book as you would any science book: Look at the table of contents and the index, read the Introduction, and then start reading the chapters. Look at the figures as you read. You'll probably be able to get through the entire book in just a couple of sittings. Then go back and reread chapters you found particularly interesting, relevant, or puzzling. Study the illustrations carefully. Pay attention to technical terminology; your instructors will use it and expect you to use it, too.

If you're a casual reader (you're not enrolled in a formal course in anatomy and physiology and have little or no background in biology), why not head to the chapters that sound the most interesting to you? Don't sweat too much over terminology; for your purposes, saying "of my lungs" communicates as well as "pulmonary." (If you also enjoy word games, though, you can get started on a whole new vocabulary.) Keep the book handy for future reference the next time you wonder what the heck they're talking about in a TV drug ad.

The 5th Wave

By Rich Tennant

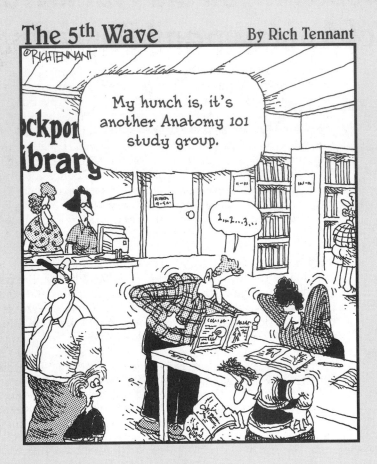

Chapter 1

Focusing on the Framework of Anatomy and Physiology

*H*uman *anatomy* is the science of the human body's structures — things that can be touched, weighed, or analyzed. Human *physiology* is the chemistry and physics of these structures, including how they all work together to support the processes of life in each individual.

If you put these two subjects together, you have the means of understanding your body on a whole new level. This chapter sets up your study of anatomy and physiology by shining a light on the very framework of the subjects, from key terminology and the levels of organization within an organism to descriptions of metabolism and homeostasis.

Looking at the Science of Anatomy and Physiology

Human anatomy and physiology are closely related to *biology*, which is the science of living beings and their relationships with the rest of the universe, including all other living beings.

If you've studied biology, you understand the basics of how organisms operate. Anatomy and physiology narrow the science of biology by looking at the specifics of one species: *Homo sapiens.*

Anatomy is structure; physiology is function. You can't talk about one without talking about the other.

Fitting anatomy and physiology into science

Biologists take for granted that human anatomy and physiology evolved from the anatomy and physiology of ancient forms. These scientists base their work on the assumption that every structure and process, no matter how tiny in scope, must somehow contribute to the survival of the individual. So each process — and the structures within which the chemistry and physics of the process actually happen — must help keep the individual alive and meeting the relentless challenges of a continually changing environment. Evolution favors processes that work.

Human *pathophysiology* is the science of "human anatomy and physiology gone wrong." (The prefix *path-* is Greek for "suffering.") It's the interface of human biology and medical science. *Clinical medicine* is the application of medical science to alleviate an anatomical or physiological problem in an individual human.

Breaking down the subsets of anatomy

The science of anatomy features the following major subsets (throughout this book, you encounter some information from each one):

- ✔ **Gross anatomy:** The study of the large parts of any animal body that can be seen with the unaided eye. (We concentrate on this aspect of anatomy in this book.)

- ✔ **Histologic anatomy:** The study of different tissue types and the cells that comprise them. Histologic anatomists use a variety of microscopes to study these cells and tissues that make up the body.

✔ **Developmental anatomy:** The study of the life cycle of the individual, from fertilized egg through adulthood, senescence (aging), and death. Body parts change throughout the life span.

✔ **Comparative anatomy:** The study of the similarities and differences among the anatomical structures of different species, including extinct species. This subject is closely related to evolutionary biology. Information from comparative anatomy helps scientists understand the human body's structures and processes. For example, the comparative anatomy of humans and living and extinct apes elucidates the structures in the human limbs that enable the bipedal posture.

Familiarizing Yourself with Anatomical Jargon

Jargon is a set of words and phrases that people who know a lot about a particular subject use to talk together. You can find jargon in every field (scientific or not), every workplace, every town, and every home. Families and close friends almost always use jargon in conversations with one another. Plumbers use jargon to communicate about plumbing. Anatomists and physiologists use jargon and technical terminology, much of which is shared with medicine and other fields of biology, especially human biology.

Scientists try to create terminology that's precise and easy to understand by developing it systematically. That is, they create new words by putting together existing and known elements. They use certain syllables or word fragments over and over to build new terms.

With a little help from this book, you can start recognizing some of these fragments. Then you can put the meanings of different fragments together and accurately guess the meaning of a term you've never seen before, just as you can understand a sentence you've never read before. Table 1-1 gets you started by listing some word fragments related to the organ systems we cover in this book.

Table 1-1   Technical Anatomical Word Fragments

Body System	Root or Word Fragment	Meaning
Skeletal system	os-, oste-	bone
	arth-	joint
Muscular system	myo-	muscle
	sarco-	flesh
Integument	derm-	skin
Nervous system	neur-	nerve
Endocrine system	aden-	gland
	estr-	steroid
Circulatory system	card-	heart (muscle)
	angi-	vessel
	hema-	blood
	arter-	artery
	ven-	venous
	erythro-	red
Respiratory system	pulmon-	lung
	bronch-	windpipe
Digestive system	gastr-	stomach
	enter-	intestine
	dent-	teeth
	hepat-	liver
Urinary system	ren-	kidney
	neph-	kidney
	ur-	urinary
Immune system	lymph-	lymph
	leuk-	white
	-itis	inflammation
Reproductive system	vagin-	vagina
	uter-	uterine

You may be asking why you should always have to parse and put back together terms like *iliohypogastric*. A key reason is the contrast between the preciseness with which scientists must name and describe the things they talk about in a scientific context and the relative vagueness and changeability of terms in plain English. Terms that people use in common speech are understood slightly differently by different people, and the meanings are always undergoing change.

Not so long ago, for example, no one speaking plain English used the term *laptop* to refer to a computer or *hybrid* to talk about a car. It's possible that, not many years from now, almost no one will understand what people meant by those words. In contrast, scientific Greek and Latin stopped changing centuries ago: *ilio, hypo,* and *gastro* have the same meanings now as they did 200 years ago.

Problems can come up when the specialists who use the jargon want to communicate with someone outside their field. The specialists must translate their message into more common terms to communicate it. Problems can also come up when someone approaching a field, such as a student, fails to make progress understanding and speaking the field's jargon. This book aims to help you make the necessary progress.

Every time you come across an anatomical or physiological term that's new to you, pull it apart to see whether any of its fragments are familiar. Using this knowledge, go as far as you can in guessing the meaning of the whole term. After studying Table 1-1, you should be able to make some pretty good guesses.

Arranging Organisms by Levels of Organization

Anatomy and physiology focus on the different levels of the *organism,* or the individual body. The life processes of the organism are built and maintained at the following several physical levels, known as *levels of organization:*

- ✔ The cellular level
- ✔ The tissue level
- ✔ The organ level
- ✔ The organ system level
- ✔ The organism level

You can see all these levels in Figure 1-1. In this section, we review these levels, starting with the smallest.

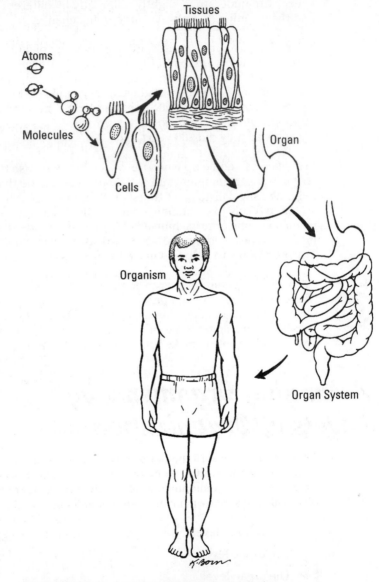

Figure 1-1: Levels of organization in the human body.

Level 1: The cellular level

If you examine a sample of any human tissue under a micro-scope, you see cells, possibly millions of cells. All living things are made of cells. In fact, having a cellular level of organiza-tion is inherent in any definition of *organism*. We discuss the cellular level of organization in some detail in Chapter 2.

Level 11: The tissue level

A *tissue* is a structure made of many cells — usually several different kinds of cells — that performs a specific function. Tissues are divided into four classes:

- **Connective tissue** serves to support body parts and bind them together.

- **Epithelial tissue** (epithelium) lines the inside of organs within the body and covers the body. The outer layer of the skin is made up of epithelial tissue.

- **Muscle tissue** is found in the muscles, which allow your body parts to move; in the walls of hollow organs to help move their contents along; and in the heart to move blood along via the acts of contraction and relaxation. (Find out more about muscles in Chapter 3.)

- **Nervous tissue** transmits impulses and forms nerves. Brain tissue is nervous tissue. (We talk about the ner-vous system in Chapter 9.)

Level 111: The organ level

An *organ* is a part of the body that performs a specialized physiological function. For example, the stomach is an organ that has the specific physiological job of breaking down food. By definition, an organ is made up of at least two different tissue types; many organs contain tissues of all four types. Although we can name and describe all four tissue types that make up all organs, as we do in the preceding section, listing all the organs in the body wouldn't be so easy.

The organs that "belong" to one system can have functions integral to another system. In fact, most organs contribute to more than one system. The blood vessels are an excellent example: They serve as a transportation network, delivering nutrients produced by the digestive system to the skeletal muscles to provide energy for locomotion and to a woman's uterus to support her developing fetus. These vessels also remove the byproducts of the energy consumed in locomotion and by the fetus in development and carry them to the organs of the urinary system for excretion.

Level IV: The organ system level

Human anatomists and physiologists have divided the human body into *organ systems,* groups of organs that work together to meet a major physiological need. For example, the digestive system is one of the organ systems responsible for obtaining energy from the environment. Other organ systems include the musculoskeletal system, the integument, and the nervous system. (The chapter structure of this book is based on the definition of organ systems.)

Level V: The organism level

This level consists of the whole enchilada — the real "you." As anatomists study organ systems, organs, tissues, and cells, they're always looking at things from the organism level.

Metabolism: Keeping Body Processes in Motion

Even when your outside is staying still, your insides are moving. Day and night, your muscles twitch and contract and maintain "tone." Your heart beats. Your blood circulates. Your diaphragm moves up and down with every breath. Nerve impulses travel. Your brain keeps tabs on everything. You think. Even when you're asleep, you dream (a form of thinking). Your intestines push the food you ate hours ago along your alimentary canal. Your kidneys filter your blood and make urine. Your sweat glands open and close. Your eyes blink, and even during sleep, they move. Men produce sperm. Women move through the menstrual cycle. The processes that keep you alive are always active.

You can thank *metabolism* — the chemical reactions occurring in the body — for keeping these many processes going. These chemical reactions consist of *anabolic reactions,* which create things (molecules), and *catabolic reactions,* which break things down. Your body performs both anabolic and catabolic reactions at the same time and around the clock to keep you alive and functioning.

To keep the meanings of anabolic and catabolic clear in your mind, associate the word *catabolic* with the word *catastrophic* to remember that catabolic reactions break down products. Then you'll know that anabolic reactions create products.

The following sections describe the reactions that your cells undergo to convert fuel to usable energy.

Seeing why your cells metabolize

Every cell in your body is like a tiny factory, converting raw materials to useful molecules, such as proteins and thousands of other products, many of which we discuss throughout this book. The raw materials (nutrients) come from the food you eat, and the cells use those nutrients in metabolic reactions. During these reactions, some of the energy from catabolized (broken down) nutrients is used to generate a compound called *adenosine triphosphate* (ATP). Whenever ATP is catabolized, it releases energy that the cell can use.

So here's how it works: Nutrients are catabolized, ATP is formed (anabolized), and ATP is catabolized when needed. This principle of linked anabolic and catabolic reactions is one of the cornerstones of human physiology and is required to maintain life. Cellular metabolism also makes waste products that must be removed (exported) from the cell and ultimately from the body.

Understanding the process behind cellular metabolism

The reactions that convert fuel to usable energy (ATP molecules) include glycolysis, aerobic respiration (the Krebs cycle), anaerobic respiration, and oxidative phosphorylation. Together these reactions are referred to as *cellular respiration*. These are complex pathways, so expect to take some time to understand them. Refer to Figure 1-2 as many times as necessary to make sure you understand what happens in cellular respiration.

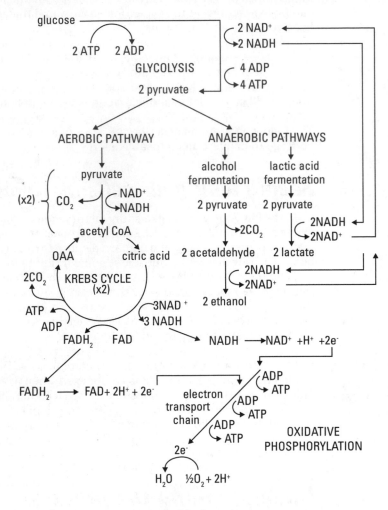

Respiration

Figure 1-2: The group of reactions that convert energy from fuel into ATP.

Glycolysis, the process that breaks down glucose, occurs in the *cytoplasm* (fluid portion) of every cell. Pyruvic acid, the product of glycolysis, moves from the cytoplasm into the cellular organelle called the *mitochondrion,* the cell's power-house. The *Krebs cycle,* also called the *tricarboxylic acid cycle* or the *citric acid cycle,* takes place in the mitochondrion.

At the completion of the Krebs cycle, the high-energy molecules that are created during the cycle move into the *membrane* of the mitochondrion, where they're passed down the electron transport chain. At the end of that chain, the molecules are used to form ATP from adenosine diphosphate (ADP) and inorganic phosphate (P_i), and water is released.

ATP is the cell's energy currency. Just as you can't keep spending money without earning some money to replenish your supply, your body can't keep expending energy without taking in more fuel. When the cell needs energy to fuel its metabolism, it pays with ATP molecules. See Figure 1-3 for the chemical structure of the ATP and related ADP molecules.

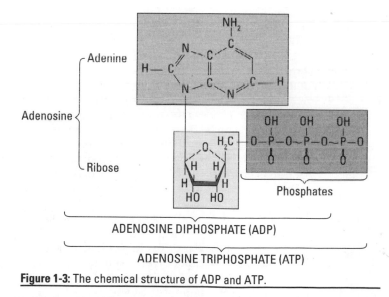

Figure 1-3: The chemical structure of ADP and ATP.

The sections that follow break down each chemical reaction that plays a role in *cellular respiration* — glycolysis, Krebs cycle, and oxidative phosphorylation.

Glycolysis

Starting at the top of Figure 1-3, you can see that glucose — the smallest molecule that a carbohydrate can be broken into during digestion — goes through the process of *glycolysis,* which starts cellular respiration and uses some energy (ATP) itself. Glycolysis occurs in the cytoplasm and doesn't require oxygen.

Two molecules of ATP are required to start each molecule of glucose rolling down the glycolytic pathway; although four molecules of ATP are generated during glycolysis, the net production of ATP is two molecules. In addition to the two ATPs, two molecules of *pyruvic acid* (also called *pyruvate*) are generated. The pyruvate molecules then move into a mitochondrion and enter the Krebs cycle.

Krebs cycle

The *Krebs cycle* is a major biological pathway in the metabolism of every multicellular organism. It's an *aerobic pathway,* requiring oxygen.

As the pyruvate enters the mitochondrion, a molecule of a compound called *nicotinamide adenine dinucleotide* (NAD+) joins it. NAD+ is an electron carrier (that is, it carries energy), and it gets the process moving by bringing some energy into the pathway. The NAD+ provides enough energy that when it joins with pyruvate, carbon dioxide is released, and the high-energy molecule NADH is formed. The product of the overall reaction is *acetyl coenzyme A* (acetyl CoA), which is a carbohydrate molecule that puts the Krebs cycle in motion.

Cycles are endless. Products of some reactions in the cycle are used to keep the cycle going. An example is acetyl CoA: It's a product of the Krebs cycle, yet it also helps initiate the cycle. With the addition of water and acetyl CoA, *oxaloacetic acid* (OAA) is converted to *citric acid.* Then, a series of reactions proceeds throughout the cycle.

Oxidative phosphorylation

Oxidative phosphorylation, which uses high energy electrons to produce ATP, is also called the *respiratory chain* and the *electron transport chain.* The electron carriers produced during the Krebs cycle — NADH and $FADH_2$ — are created when NAD+ and FAD, respectively, are reduced. When a substance is *reduced,* it gains electrons; when it's *oxidized,* it loses electrons.

So NADH and $FADH_2$ are compounds that have gained electrons and, therefore, energy. In the respiratory chain, oxidation and reduction reactions occur repeatedly as a way of transporting energy. At the end of the chain, oxygen atoms accept the electrons, producing water. (Water from metabolic reactions isn't a significant contributor to the water needs of the body.)

As NADH and $FADH_2$ pass down the respiratory (or electron transport) chain, they lose energy as they become oxidized and reduced, oxidized and reduced, oxidized and. . . . It sounds exhausting, doesn't it? Well, their energy supplies become exhausted for a good cause.

The energy that these electron carriers lose is used to add a molecule of phosphorus to adenosine *di*phosphate (ADP) to make it adenosine *tri*phosphate — the coveted ATP. And ATP is the goal for converting the energy in food to energy that the cells in the body can use. For each NADH molecule that's produced in the Krebs cycle, three molecules of ATP can be generated. For each molecule of $FADH_2$ that's produced in the Krebs cycle, two molecules of ATP are made.

Theoretically, the entire process of aerobic cellular respiration — glycolysis, Krebs cycle, and oxidative phosphorylation — generates a total of 38 ATP molecules from the energy in one molecule of glucose: 2 from glycolysis, 2 from the Krebs cycle, and 34 from oxidative phosphorylation. However, this theoretical yield is never quite reached because processes, especially biological processes, are never 100 percent efficient. In the real world, usually around 29 to 30 ATP molecules per glucose molecule are expected.

Anaerobic respiration

Sometimes oxygen isn't present, but your body still needs energy. During these rare times, a backup system, an *anaerobic pathway* (called *anaerobic* because it proceeds in the absence of oxygen) exists. Lactic acid fermentation generates NAD+ so that glycolysis, which results in the production of two molecules of ATP, can continue. However, if the supply of NAD+ runs out, glycolysis can't occur, and ATP can't be generated.

Balancing Bodily Reactions with Homeostasis

Chemical reactions aren't random events. Any reaction takes place only when all the conditions are right for it: All the required reagents and catalysts are close together in the right quantities; the fuel for the reaction is present, in sufficient amount and in the right form; and the environmental variables are all within the right range, including the temperature, salinity, and pH.

The complicated chemistry of life is extremely sensitive to the environmental conditions; the environment is the body itself. *Homeostasis* is the term physiologists use to mean the subset of metabolic reactions that keep the internal environment of the body in a state conducive to the chemical reactions that maintain your life.

The following sections look at a few important physiological variables and how the mechanisms of homeostasis keep them in the optimum range in common, everyday situations.

Because homeostatic reactions are metabolic actions, they require energy.

Regulating body temperature

All metabolic reactions in all organisms require that the temperature of the body be within a certain range. But humans, the land-loving creatures that they are, are often subjected to large and sudden temperature changes in their environments.

The key solution to this problem is called *homeothermy,* or warm-bloodedness, which is described as the maintenance of body temperature at a relatively constant level regardless of the ambient temperature. The large number of mitochondria per cell that humans possess enables a high rate of metabolism, which in turn generates a lot of heat. Warm-blooded animals must ingest a large quantity of food frequently to fuel their higher metabolism.

Regulating body temperature requires a steady supply of fuel (glucose) to the mitochondrial furnaces.

Another way warm-blooded animals control their body temperatures is by employing adaptations that conserve the heat generated by metabolism within the body in cold conditions or dissipate that heat out of the body in overly warm conditions. A few of the specific adaptations humans use to hold their internal temperatures constant are

- ✔ **Sweating:** Sweat glands in the skin open to dissipate heat by evaporative cooling of water from the skin. They close to conserve heat. Sweat glands are opened and closed by the actions of muscles at the base of the gland deep under the skin.

- ✔ **Blood circulation:** Blood vessels close to the skin dilate (enlarge) to dissipate heat in the blood through the skin. They constrict (narrow) to conserve heat. Your skin flushes (reddens) when you're hot because that's the color of your blood visible at the surface of your skin.

- ✔ **Muscle contraction:** When sweating and blood vessel constriction aren't enough to conserve heat in cold conditions, your muscles begin to contract automatically to generate more heat. This reaction is often referred to as *shivering*.

- ✔ **Insulation:** Mammals and birds evolved insulating structures on their body surfaces (hair and feathers, respectively) and regions of fatty tissue under the skin. Humans alone employ the cultural adaptation of clothing.

Maintaining a fluid balance

A watery environment is part of the requirements for a great proportion of metabolic reactions. (The rest need a lipid, or fatty, environment.) The body contains a lot of water. You have water in your blood, in your cells, in the spaces between your cells, in your digestive organs, here, there, and everywhere. Not pure water, though. The water in your body is a solvent for thousands of different ions and molecules (solutes). The quantity and quality of the solutes change the character of the solution.

Because solutes are constantly entering and leaving the solution as they participate in or are generated by metabolic reactions, the characteristics of the watery solution must remain within certain bounds for the reactions to continue. The following fluid-balance homeostasis mechanisms have evolved:

✓ **The thirst reflex:** Water passes through your body constantly: mainly, in through your mouth and out through various organ systems, including the skin, the digestive system, and the urinary system. If the volume of water falls below the optimum level (resulting in dehydration), the mechanisms of homeostasis intrude on your conscious brain to make you uncomfortable. You feel thirsty. You ingest something watery. Your fluid balance is restored, and your thirst reflex leaves you alone.

✓ **The ability to change the composition of urine:** The kidney is a complex organ that has the ability to measure the concentration of many solutes in the blood, including sodium, potassium, and calcium. The kidney can measure the volume of water in the body by sensing the pressure of the blood as it flows through. The greater the volume of water, the higher the blood pressure.

If changes must be made to bring the volume and composition of the blood back into the ideal range, the various structures of the kidney incorporate more or less water, sodium, potassium, and so on into the urine. This process explains why your urine is paler or darker at different times.

Examining blood glucose concentration

Glucose, the fuel of all cellular processes, is distributed to all cells dissolved in the blood. The concentration of glucose in the blood must be high enough to ensure that the cells have enough fuel. However, extra glucose beyond the immediate needs of the cells can harm many important organs and tissues, especially where the vessels are tiny, as in the retina of the eye, the extremities (hands and, especially, feet), and the kidneys.

The amount of glucose in the blood is controlled mainly by the intestines and by insulin. *Insulin* is a hormone released from the pancreas, an endocrine gland, into the blood in response to increased blood glucose levels.

Most cells have receptors that bind the insulin, which increases the activity of glucose transporters in the cell membrane. Glucose is removed from the blood and into storage, mostly within the cells of the liver, the muscles (where it's stored as glycogen, the form of fuel your muscles use), and the fat cells of the adipose tissue. At times when your intestines aren't releasing much glucose, such as some hours after a meal, the production of insulin is suppressed, and the stored glucose is released into the blood again.

Gauging variables that keep the body balanced

How does the pancreas know when to release insulin and how much is enough? How does the kidney know when the salt content of the blood is too high or the volume of the blood is too low? What tells the sweat glands to open and close to cool the body or retain heat? The answer in these and many other situations related to homeostasis is this: The detection of threats to homeostasis and the response of organs to counter the threats involve an intricate system of communications between parts of the nervous, circulatory, and endocrine systems.

Here's the general process of how this communication works:

1. **Receptors (sensors) in the blood vessels detect the state of the blood.**

   Some receptors detect temperature, some pressure (volume), some the concentration of glucose, and many others detect different variables.

2. **The receptors send their data through the nervous system to the brain, where an endocrine gland called the *hypothalamus* resides.**

   The hypothalamus is sometimes called the *master gland* because it controls homeostasis by acting on other glands, notably the *pituitary gland.*

3. **The endocrine system makes and releases hormones that travel through the blood to the tissues and organs and cause them to change their behavior in ways that restore the variables to their optimum physiological range.**

   Hormones are substances of great power and subtlety.

Chapter 2

Examining Cell Biology Basics

· ·

· ·

*B*iologists see life as existing at five levels of organization, of which the cellular level is the first (see Chapter 1 for more on the levels of organization). A basic principle of biology says that all organisms are made of cells and that anything that has even one cell is an organism. Understanding the basics of cell biology is necessary for understanding any aspect of biology, including human anatomy and physiology.

This chapter clues you in to cell biology basics so you have some context for the various physiological processes we describe in later chapters.

How Cells Spend Their Time

Almost all the structures of anatomy are built of cells, and almost all the functions of physiology are carried out in cells. A comprehensive list of cell functions would be impossible, but we can group cell functions into a few main categories, which we do in the following sections.

Creating new cells

Cells arise from other cells and nowhere else. Once in an organism's lifetime, at the beginning, two cells fuse to form a new cell. As a result, all the cells in an organism's lifetime ultimately derive from the first one.

This process is how an organism builds itself from one single generic cell to a complex organism comprising trillions of highly differentiated, highly specialized, and highly efficient cells all working together in a coordinated way. Here's a look at how a cell goes from one to many.

- ✓ **Fusing:** The organism's first cell is the *zygote,* made by the fusion of sex cells: an *ovum* (egg cell) from the female parent and a *sperm* cell from the male parent.

- ✓ **Dividing:** In the form of cell division called *mitosis,* one cell divides into two *daughter cells,* each of them complete but smaller than the original cell.

- ✓ **Differentiating:** After mitosis is complete, each daughter cell goes on to its own separate life. One or both may start or continue down a path of *differentiation,* the name for processes that give cells their particular structures and functions. A cell destined to become a nerve cell starts down one path of differentiation; a cell destined to become a muscle cell starts down another path.

Manufacturing tissues

All tissues are made of and built by cells and are maintained by them, too. Cells in a tissue are, to one degree or another, *differentiated* or *specialized* for their anatomical or physiological function in the tissue.

For the purposes of anatomy and physiology, keep in mind that all cells have some important features in common, but they also differentiate into a vast array of shapes and sizes, containing vastly diverse structures and having different functions and life cycles.

Constructing and moving products

A great many types of cells make special chemicals that are incorporated into tissues and participate in metabolic reactions. Cellular products include thousands of specific proteins and polypeptides, signaling chemicals such as neurotransmitters and hormones, small molecules and ions, lipids of many kinds, and many types of cellular matrices.

Some cells specialize in transporting the products of other cells around the body or in transporting metabolic waste products out of the body. Some of these transporting cells have other functions as well. Others do nothing but that one job through their entire life cycle. Red blood cells are an extreme example of the one-job model. They lose their nuclei during differentiation and thereafter do nothing but transport gas molecules from one place to another.

Transmitting signals around the body

Some cells transmit various signals while remaining in one place in the body. Some nerve cells perform only the functions of generating and conducting electrical signals and maintaining themselves, and they typically live for years, or even until the death of the organism itself. Other cells produce various signaling molecules, such as hormones and neurotransmitters, or receive and react to those signaling molecules.

Exploring Eukaryotic Cells

Although they're astoundingly varied, cells are also remarkably alike. All cells, at least all *eukaryotic* cells, are alike. Plants, animals, and fungi are *eukaryotes* (organisms made up of eukaryotic cells), and all their cells, in all their enormous complexity and variation, are fundamentally alike.

Here's a simplistic description of a eukaryotic cell: It's a membrane-bound sac containing smaller but distinctive structures, called *organelles* ("little organs"), suspended in a gel like matrix called *cytoplasm*. As their name suggests, organelles are functional subunits of a cell, just as organs are functional subunits of an organism.

Figure 2-1 shows the general structure of a eukaryotic cell. Refer to this figure as you read about the various cellular structures in the following sections. Table 2-1 gives an overview of the structures found within a eukaryotic cell.

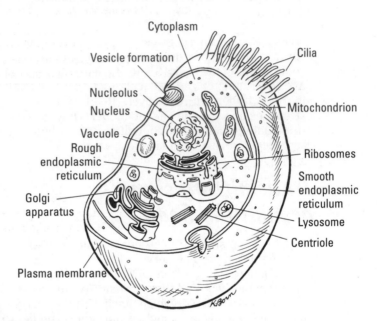

Figure 2-1: A cutaway view of a basic animal cell and its organelles.

Table 2-1	Organelles of All Animal Cells
Organelle	*Function*
Nucleus	Controls the cell; houses the genetic material
Mitochondrion	Cell powerhouse
Endoplasmic reticulum	Plays an important role in protein synthesis; participates in transporting cell products; involved in metabolizing fats
Ribosome	Binds amino acids together under the direction of mRNA to make protein

Organelle	Function
Golgi apparatus	Packages cellular products in sacs called vesicles so some of the products can cross the cell membrane to exit the cell
Vacuoles	Membrane-bound spaces in the cytoplasm that sometimes serve in the active transport of materials to the cell membrane for discharge to the outside of the cell
Lysosomes	Contain digestive enzymes that break down harmful cell products and waste materials and actively transport them out of the cell

Enclosing it all with the cell membrane

A cell is bound by the *cell membrane* (also called the *plasma membrane*). The cell membrane of all eukaryotes is made of *phospholipid* molecules. These molecules are made by cells, a process that requires energy. The molecules assemble spontaneously (without input of energy) into the membrane, obeying the forces of *polarity*.

The structure of the cell membrane and the various proteins inserted in it is important for cell function.

Explaining the fluid-mosaic model

The phospholipid bilayer is embedded with structures of many different kinds. Though the bilayer itself is essentially similar in all cells, the embedded structures are as various and specialized as the cells themselves. Some structures identify the cell to other cells (which is important in immune system functioning), and others control the movement of certain substances in or out of the cell across the membrane.

Figure 2-2 is a diagrammatic representation of the phospholipid bilayer and embedded structures. This model of the cell membrane is called the *fluid-mosaic model. Fluid* describes the ability of molecules in the bilayer to move; *mosaic* pertains to the embedded structures.

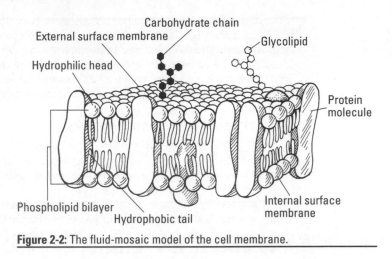

Carbohydrate chain
External surface membrane
Glycolipid
Hydrophilic head
Protein molecule
Phospholipid bilayer
Hydrophobic tail
Internal surface membrane

Figure 2-2: The fluid-mosaic model of the cell membrane.

The chemical properties of the phospholipid bilayer and the embedded structures contribute to an important feature of the cell membrane: It controls which substances pass through it and which don't. This control means the membrane is *semipermeable.*

Moving across the membrane passively

Some substances, mainly small molecules and ions, cross the membrane by a *passive transport* mechanism, meaning they more or less flow unimpeded across the bilayer, driven by the forces of ordinary chemistry, such as concentration gradients, random molecular movement, and polarity.

Here are some ways that substances cross a membrane passively:

- ✔ **Diffusion:** A substance moves spontaneously down a *concentration gradient* (from a highly concentrated area to a less concentrated area). For example, if you drop a teaspoon of salt into a jar of water, the dissolved sodium and chloride ions will, in time, *diffuse* (spread themselves evenly through the water).

- ✔ **Osmosis:** The diffusion of water molecules across a selectively permeable membrane gets a special name: *osmosis.*

✔ **Filtration:** This form of passive transport occurs during capillary exchange. (*Capillaries* are the smallest blood vessels that bridge arterioles and venules; see Chapter 4 for details on the circulatory system.) Capillaries are only one cell layer thick, and the capillary cell membrane acts as a filter, controlling the entrance and exit of small molecules.

Passing through the membrane actively

Active transport allows a cell to control which big, active, biological molecules move in and out of the cytoplasm. Active transport is a fundamental characteristic of living cells.

Like many matters in cell biology, active transport mechanisms are numerous and widely varied. A simple active import mechanism has a molecule outside the cell, which helps the cell function, as well as a membrane-embedded structure that can identify the molecule with unerring specificity. The membrane-embedded structure frequently uses a kind of lock-and-key mechanism and can communicate its presence to another membrane-embedded structure. The second structure then opens a channel that only the specific molecule can pass through, and the channel closes until the structure gets another reliable message to open up.

A slightly more complex variation of the preceding process involves a transport molecule that brings the molecule from the cell where it was made to the cell where it's used.

Relinquishing control to the nucleus

The defining characteristic of a eukaryotic cell is the presence of a nucleus, which directs the cell's activity. The largest organelle, the nucleus is oval or round and is plainly visible under a microscope. Refer to Figure 2-1 to see the relationship of the nucleus to the cell.

Giving the organelles a place to hang in the cytoplasm

Within the cell membrane, between and around the organelles, is a fluid matrix called *cytoplasm* (or *cytosol*). The cytoplasm also contains internal scaffolding made of *microfilaments* and *microtubules* that support the cell, give processes the space they need, and protect the organelles. The organelles are suspended in the cytoplasm.

Seeing how mitochondria provide energy to cells

A *mitochondrion* (plural, *mitochondria*) is an organelle that transforms energy into a form that can be used to fuel the cell's metabolism and functions. It's often called the cell's *powerhouse.* We describe the role of the mitochondrion in cellular respiration in Chapter 1.

The number of mitochondria in a cell depends on the cell's function. Cells whose function requires only a little energy, such as nerve cells, have relatively few mitochondria; muscle cells may contain several thousand individual mitochondria because of their function in using energy to do work. A mitochondrion can divide, like a cell, to produce more mitochondria, and it can grow, move, and combine with other mitochondria, all to support the cell's need for energy.

Producing protein in the endoplasmic reticulum (ER)

The process of protein construction begins in the nucleus. In response to many different kinds of signals, certain genes become active, setting off the production of a specific protein molecule (gene expression). Think of the nucleus as a factory's administrative department.

The *endoplasmic reticulum* (or ER) is a chain of membrane-bound canals and cavities that runs in a convoluted path, connecting the cell membrane with the nuclear envelope. The ER brings all the components required for protein synthesis together. Think of the ER as a factory's logistics function.

The *ribosomes* are the site of protein synthesis where the binding reactions that build a chain of amino acids are performed. Ribosomes are organelles that may float in the cytoplasm or adhere to the outer surface of some parts of the ER membrane, sticking out into the cytoplasm. These areas are called *rough ER* (in contrast to *smooth ER,* where no ribosomes adhere). Ribosomes are tiny, even by the standard of organelles, but they're highly energetic, and a typical cell contains thousands of them. Think of the ribosomes as the production machinery.

The *Golgi body* forms a part of the *cellular endomembrane system,* which includes the nuclear membrane and the ER. It functions in the storage, modification, and secretion of proteins and lipids. Think of it as the shipping department of a factory.

Taking out the trash with lysosomes

Old, worn-out cell parts need to be removed from the cells; if they aren't, they can become sources of toxins or severe energy drains. *Lysosomes* are organelles that do the dirty work of *autodigestion.* Lysosomal enzymes destroy another part of the cell, say an old mitochondrion, through a digestive process. Molecules that can be recovered from the mitochondrion are recycled in that cell or in another. Waste products are excreted from the cell in a membrane-bound vacuole.

Macromolecules, the Building Blocks of Life

Macromolecules, molecules that are many thousands of times larger than water or carbon dioxide, are constructed in cells and react together in seemingly miraculous ways. These building blocks of life — nucleic acids (DNA and RNA), polysaccharides, and proteins — are all made mainly of carbon, with varying proportions of oxygen, hydrogen, nitrogen, and phosphorous.

Macromolecules are made of molecular subunits called, generically, *monomers* ("one piece"); each type of macromolecule has its own kind of monomer. Macromolecules are, therefore, *polymers* ("many pieces").

The following sections focus on these large molecules and their complex interactions. The amazing chemistry of these polymeric macromolecules is the chemistry of life.

Naming the nucleic acids and nucleotides

The nucleic acids *DNA* (deoxyribonucleic acid) and *RNA* (ribonucleic acid) are polymers that are made of monomers called *nucleotides* and are arranged in chains one after another. And another and another. . . . Although both DNA and RNA molecules are long, DNA molecules are thousands of nucleotides long. The functioning of genes is inseparable from the chemical structure of the nucleic acid monomers.

The structural similarities and differences between DNA and RNA allow them to work together to produce proteins within cells. The DNA molecule remains stable in the nucleus during normal cell functioning and is protected from damage by the nuclear envelope. An RNA molecule is built on demand to transmit a gene's coded instructions for building proteins, and then it disintegrates. Some of its nucleotide subunits remain intact and are recycled into new RNA molecules.

Energizing organisms with polysaccharides

The simple carbohydrate molecule called *glucose* is the main energy molecule in physiology. *Polysaccharides,* which are polymers of carbohydrate monomers like glucose, are useful in animal physiology, including human physiology, as fuel storage (glycogen).

Polysaccharides play more roles in plant, fungal, and bacterial physiology by forming much of the (connective) structural tissue, a role taken largely by proteins in animals. However, polysaccharides are as vital (required for life) for animals as they are for plants.

Peeking at proteins

Proteins, also called *polypeptides,* are polymers of *amino acids.* The amino acid monomers are arranged in a linear chain and may be folded and refolded into a globular form. Structural proteins comprise about 75 percent of your body's material. The integument, the muscles, the joints, and the other kinds of connective tissue are made mostly of structural proteins, such as collagen, keratin, actin, and myosin. In addition, the *enzymes* that catalyze all the complex chemical reactions of life in all organisms (plants, fungi, bacteria, and animals) are also proteins.

Amino acids

Twenty different amino acids exist in nature. Amino acids themselves are, by the standards of nonliving chemistry, huge and complex. A typical protein comprises hundreds of amino acid monomers that must be attached in exactly the right order for the protein to function properly.

Enzymes

Enzymes are protein molecules that *catalyze,* or change, the chemical reactions of life. Enzymes can only speed up a reaction that's otherwise chemically possible. How effective are enzymes in speeding up reactions? A reaction that may take a century or more to happen spontaneously happens in a fraction of a second with the right enzyme.

Enzymes are involved in every physiological process, and each enzyme is extremely specific to one or a few individual reactions. Your body has tens of thousands of different enzymes.

Discovering How Genetic Material Makes You Who You Are

Your anatomical structures are specified in detail, and all your physiological processes are controlled by your own unique set of *genes.* Unless you're an identical twin, this particular set of genes, called your *genome,* is yours alone, created at the moment your mother's ovum and your father's sperm fused. The genome itself is incorporated in the DNA in the nucleus of every one of your cells.

Your genes are responsible for your *traits.* If your genes specify that you'll grow to 6 feet tall (a trait), they cause bone and tissue to grow until your body reaches that height, and they maintain it thereafter (assuming a favorable environment), until the cells the genes work through age and die. Similarly, if you have the genes for brown eyes (a trait), your genes direct the production of pigments that color the eyes.

How do genes actually produce your traits? A gene that's active sends messages to its own cell or to other cells, ordering them to produce molecules of its particular protein, the only one it's capable of making. The message is sent from DNA through the intermediary of *mRNA* (messenger RNA), which places an order at the protein factory of the cell and stays around for a while to supervise production. This process is referred to as *gene expression.*

Here's a brief rundown of the three parts of the process:

- ✓ **Transcription:** The first part of the process, where DNA writes the order in the form of a sequence of nucleotides on mRNA, takes place in the nucleus and is called *transcription* ("writing across").

- ✓ **Translation:** The next part of the process, where RNA places the order at the protein factory of the cell, is called *translation* ("carrying across").

- ✓ **Posttranslational modifications:** The last part, where the amino acid monomers are sorted out and assembled into the polypeptide, starts in the ribosome. The finishing touches are put on the protein molecule in the endoplasmic reticulum and the Golgi body.

Cycling through Life, Cell-Style

The life cycle of an individual cell is called the *cell cycle.* The moment of *cell cleavage,* when a cell membrane grows across the "equator" of a dividing cell, is considered to be the end of the cycle for the mother cell and the beginning of the cycle for the daughter cells. We walk you through the phases of the cell cycle in the following sections.

Progressing through interphase

Interphase begins when the cell membrane fully encloses the new cell and lasts until the beginning of mitosis or meiosis. The duration of interphase may be anywhere from minutes to decades.

Generally speaking (exceptions always exist in cell biology), cells do most of their differentiating and most of their routine metabolizing during interphase. Stem cells grow in size and reduplicate organelles during interphase, in preparation for mitosis. Some other cells enter mitosis after an extended period of steady-state metabolism. Sometimes, a cell remains in interphase, carrying out its physiological function for years and years until it dies.

Pushing ahead to DNA replication

DNA replication is an early event in cell division, occurring during interphase, just prior to the beginning of mitosis or meiosis but within the protected space in the nuclear envelope. Maintaining the integrity of the DNA code is vital.

During DNA replication, the double helix must untwist and "unzip" so the two strands of DNA are split apart. As shown in Figure 2-3, each strand becomes a template for building the new complementary strand. This process occurs a little at a time along a strand of DNA. The entire DNA strand doesn't unravel and split apart all at once. When the top part of the helix is open, the original DNA strand looks like a Y. This partly open/partly closed area where replication occurs is the *replication fork.*

Entering mitosis

A cell enters a process of *mitosis* (division) in response to signals from the nucleus. As you can see in Figure 2-4, mitosis is a multistage process.

When each of the two identical nuclei is at opposite poles of the cell, mitosis is technically over. However, the cell's cytoplasm still has to split into two masses, a process called *cytokinesis.* The center of the mother cell indents and squeezes the cell membrane across the cytoplasm until two separate cells are formed. The two daughter cells are then in interphase. At this point, they may go on to differentiation, depending on the instructions to the cell from the genome.

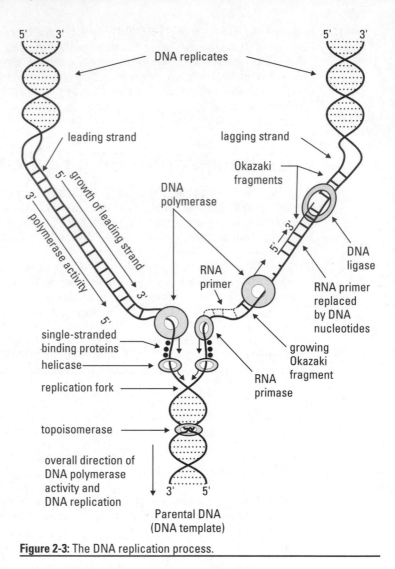

Figure 2-3: The DNA replication process.

 All cells arise from the division of another cell, but not all cells go on to divide again. The following list describes cells that divide and some that don't:

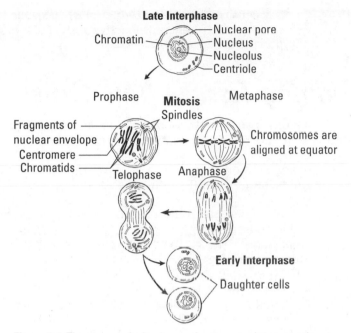

Figure 2-4: The stages of mitosis: prophase, metaphase, anaphase, and telophase.

✔ **Zygote:** The *zygote* is the diploid cell that comes into existence when the sex cells (ovum and sperm, both haploid) fuse at conception. Almost immediately, the zygote divides into two somatic cells.

✔ **Somatic cells:** The *somatic cells* include all the cells of the body except the sex cells. Somatic cells may be *relatively differentiated* (somewhat specialized) or *terminally differentiated* (they never divide again), or they may be stem cells.

✔ **Stem cells:** *Stem cells* are special kinds of generic somatic cells that divide to produce one new stem cell and one new somatic cell that goes on to differentiate into a particular type of cell in a particular type of tissue.

An *embryo* (an organism in the early stages of development) has special stem cells, called *pluripotent* ("many powers") stem cells, which have the ability to give rise to just about any kind of cell an organism needs, given the right chemical environment.

> ✓ **Sex cells (gametes):** *Sex cells* form when specialized somatic cells in the reproductive system divide by a process called *meiosis.*

Forming Tissues from Cells

A *tissue* is an assemblage of cells, not necessarily identical but from the same origin, that together carry out a specific function. As you discover in Chapter 1, tissue is the second level of organization in organisms, above (larger than) the cell level and below (smaller than) the organ level.

Like just about everything else in anatomy, tissues are many and various, and they're grouped into a reasonable number of types to make talking about them and understanding them a little simpler. The tissues of the animal body are grouped into four types: *connective tissue, epithelial tissue, muscle tissue,* and *nervous tissue.* All body tissues are classified into one of these groups. We explain the first two in the following sections. We cover muscle and nervous tissue in Chapters 3 and 9, respectively.

Linking structures with connective tissue

Connective tissues connect, support, and bind body structures together. Generally, connective tissue is made of cells that are spaced far apart within a gel-like, semisolid, solid, or fluid matrix. (A *matrix* is a material that surrounds and supports cells. In a chocolate chip cookie, for example, the dough is the matrix for the chocolate chips.)

Connective tissue has many functions, and thus many forms. In some parts of the body, such as the bones, connective tissue supports the weight of other structures, which may or may not be directly connected to it. Other connective tissue, such as adipose tissue (fat pads), cushions other structures from impact. Every organ system in the human body has some kind of connective tissue.

Aside from bones and cartilage (see Chapter 3) and blood (see Chapter 4), other types of connective tissue found in the human body are

✔ **Areolar tissue:** This loose connective tissue surrounds and separates structures in every part of the body.

✔ **Dense regular connective tissue:** The secretory cells of this type of connective tissue produce dense bands and sheets of parallel protein fibers, such as those in ligaments and tendons.

✔ **Dense irregular connective tissue:** The protein fibers in this tissue type are arranged in thick, tough, irregularly oriented bundles.

✔ **Adipose tissue:** Composed of fat cells, this loose connective tissue provides fuel storage as well as support and protection to its underlying structures.

✔ **Reticular tissue:** This type of loose connective tissue forms a web and functions as a filter in such organs as the spleen, the lymph nodes, and the bone marrow.

Reviewing types of epithelial tissue

Epithelial tissue forms the epidermis of the *integument* (the skin and the accessory structures such as sweat glands, oil glands, nails, and hair follicles), a continuous covering of the outside of the body (described in Chapter 3), and the *endothelium*, a continuous lining of the internal surfaces of the blood vessels. Epithelial tissue comes in ten types; each one is defined by the way epithelial cells are combined and shaped (see Figure 2-5).

✔ **Simple squamous epithelium:** This tissue, a single layer of flat cells, functions in rapid diffusion and filtration.

✔ **Simple cuboidal epithelium:** This tissue, which is a single layer of cuboidal cells, functions in absorption and secretion. It's typically found in glands.

✔ **Simple columnar epithelium:** This tissue is made of a single layer of cells that are elongated in one dimension (like a column) and usually densely packed. Like simple cuboidal epithelium, this tissue functions in secretion and absorption.

✔ **Simple columnar ciliated epithelium:** This tissue possesses a type of organelle called *cilia* — hairlike structures that act to move substances along in waves.

✔ **Pseudostratified columnar epithelium:** This tissue is made from a single layer of columnar cells. Note that the prefix *pseudo* means "false." The tissue appears stratified, or layered, because the cells' nuclei don't line up in a row as they do in simple columnar epithelium.

✔ **Pseudostratified columnar ciliated epithelium:** These cells are the same as the pseudostratified columnar epithelium, but they also feature cilia.

✔ **Stratified squamous epithelium:** This tissue consists of several layers of cells — squamous epithelial cells on the outside with deeper layers of cuboidal or columnar epithelial cells. It's found in areas where the outer layer is subject to wear and needs to be replaced continuously.

✔ **Stratified cuboidal epithelium:** This tissue is made of several layers of cuboidal cells that mainly act as protection.

✔ **Stratified columnar epithelium:** This tissue is a multilayered absorptive and secretive tissue.

✔ **Transitional epithelium:** The cells of this tissue can change (or *transition*) from dome-shaped or scalloped-shaped to squamous (flat) and back again, as needed by the tissue.

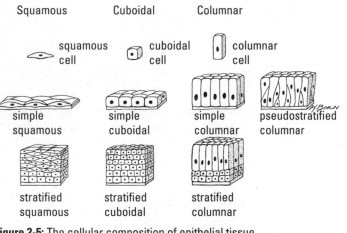

Figure 2-5: The cellular composition of epithelial tissue.

Chapter 3

Scoping Out the Body's Structural Layers

● ●

In This Chapter

▶ Discovering the functions of your skeleton

▶ Understanding your muscular system

▶ Appreciating your skin, hair, and nails

● ●

*Y*ou're not an amorphous blob of cells. The things that give your body its form, allow it to move, and protect it are the *structural layers*. Following are the three main structural components in the body:

✔ **The skeletal system:** The skeleton determines the general shape and size of humans as a species. In humans, as in all vertebrates, the skeleton is part of the *musculoskeletal system.*

✔ **The muscular system:** Muscle tissues work together with all the other systems in your body, but more than any other organ system, the muscular systems specialize in movement.

✔ **The integumentary system:** The skin and its appendages (hair and nails), together called the *integument,* make up the body's largest organ system.

This chapter shows you what your skeleton, muscle, and skin are made of and explains how they're organized.

The Skinny on Your Skeleton

The structural functions of the skeletal system are

✓ **Protection:** Bones and joints are strong and resilient, so they shelter and protect your organs. For example, the rib cage provides a protected inner space for your more delicate internal organs. The vertebral column partially encases and protects the spinal cord, and the skull completely encases the brain.

✓ **Movement:** The musculoskeletal system is a motion machine: The bones anchor the skeletal muscles and act as levers, the joints act as fulcrums, and muscle contraction provides the force for movement.

✓ **Support:** The curved vertebral column supports most of your body's weight. The arches of your feet support the weight of your body in a different way.

Examining the skeleton's makeup

This section explains how your body builds the tissues of the bones and the joints and describes how they all fit together to protect, move, and support the entire body.

Connective tissue

The skeleton is made up of three types of connective tissue:

✓ **Bone tissue** is physiologically active, is constantly generating and repairing itself, and has a generous blood supply running through it. It also makes a huge amount of cells that are exported to the rest of the body, notably the very cells of the blood. Bone tissue contains dozens of specialized cell types, and all the skeletal system's functions depend on the functioning of specialized cells in the tissue.

✓ **Cartilage** is a firm but flexible tissue that's made up of mostly protein fibers and serves as the main component of joints. Among the functions of cartilage tissue is the building of new bone. The two types of cartilage in the skeletal system are hyaline cartilage and fibrocartilage.

- *Hyaline cartilage* is the type that forms the septum of your nose. It also forms a portion of the very first version of the fetal skeleton. It's the most abundant type of cartilage in several kinds of joints. For example, it's a major component of the freely movable joints called *synovial joints.*

- *Fibrocartilage* is a fibrous, spongy tissue that acts as a shock absorber in the vertebral column (spine) and the pelvis.

Cartilage isn't generated and replaced as actively as bone, so cartilage gets by with fewer cells. Mature cartilage has no blood supply.

✔ **Fibrous connective tissue** contains very few living cells and is composed mainly of protein fibers, complex sugars, and water. It forms a structure called the *periosteum,* which is a protective sheet that covers bones. The sheet morphs into cordlike structures, called *ligaments* and *tendons,* wherever necessary. Ligaments connect a bone to another bone, and tendons connect a muscle to a bone.

The periosteum is said to be *continuous* with the ligaments and tendons, because no real separation exists between the "sheet" and the "cords."

Bone structure

The structures called *bones* (such as the femur, the vertebrae, and the finger bones) are made of bone tissue. (No surprise there. However, note that the structures called *joints* are made of tissue called *cartilage.*) Remember that individual types of bones have different forms of bone tissue.

Long bones, such as your thighbone (femur) or forearm bone (radius), are the type of bones people usually think of first. And in fact, they make good illustrations of the general anatomy and physiology of bone tissue (see Figure 3-1). You can read about long bones and the other types of bones in the later section "Bone names and characteristics."

In cross section, bone is structured in concentric layers. In other words, an outer layer surrounds a middle layer, which in turn surrounds an inner layer. In longitudinal section, a bone has two (mostly similar) ends and a long middle area, which has cells and tissues that are mostly different from the ends. The following list names and briefly describes cellular and material composition of the areas of a long bone:

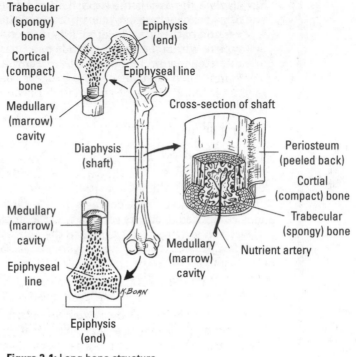

Trabecular (spongy) bone

Cortical (compact) bone

Medullary (marrow) cavity

Epiphysis (end)

Epiphyseal line

Diaphysis (shaft)

Cross-section of shaft

Periosteum (peeled back)

Cortial (compact) bone

Trabecular (spongy) bone

Nutrient artery

Medullary (marrow) cavity

Medullary (marrow) cavity

Epiphyseal line

Epiphysis (end)

K.BORN

Figure 3-1: Long bone structure.

✔ **Compact bone** (the outer layer) is a dense layer of cells in a hard matrix of protein fibers and compounds made of calcium and other minerals. This layer gives bones their amazing strength.

✔ **Spongy bone** (the middle layer) is, like compact bone, a variety of cell types within a matrix of mineralized protein fibers. But spongy bone is more open in structure than compact bone, creating a physiological trade-off between strength and lightness. Structures called *trabeculae,* which follow stress lines in the bone, act like braces, providing support.

✔ **The medullary cavity and bone marrow** is the inner layer in the shaft of a long bone (the *diaphysis*) and the inner layer of other bones. Bones have both *yellow marrow,* which is mostly fat (think butter), and *red marrow,* the site of *hematopoiesis,* which is the production of blood cells.

✔ **Epiphysis** is the enlarged, knobby end of a long bone. It consists of a layer of spongy bone covered by an outer layer of compact bone. The epiphysis is the site of bone elongation. Within the epiphysis, bone and cartilage tissue are intimately connected: As cartilage cells divide, cartilage morphs into bone tissue. This process continues from before birth until the bones reach their full adult size.

Bone names and characteristics

Bones come in different shapes and sizes. Appropriately, many bone type names match what they look like, such as flat bones, long bones, short bones, and irregular bones. Check out Table 3-1 for the differences among the four types of bones.

Table 3-1	Characteristics of Bone Types	
Bone Type	**Example Location in the Body**	**Characteristics**
Flat	Skull, shoulder blades, ribs, sternum, pelvic bones	Like plates of armor, flat bones protect soft tissues of the brain and organs in the thorax and pelvis.
Long	Arms and legs	Like steel beams, these weight-bearing bones provide structural support.
Short	Wrists (carpal bones) and ankles (tarsal bones)	Short bones look like blocks and allow a wider range of movement than larger bones.
Irregular	Vertebral column, kneecaps	Irregular bones have a variety of shapes and usually have projections that muscles, tendons, and ligaments can attach to.

Surveying joints and their movements

A *joint* is a connection between two bones. Some joints move freely, some move little, and some never move. Joints, which vary greatly in their size and shape, are classified by the amount of movement they permit. The following sections tell you about the different joint structures and what they allow you to do.

Categorizing the types of joints

The human skeleton features the following three types of joints, and they all provide a different range of motion:

- ✓ **Immovable joints:** Joints that don't move, such as those between the bones of the skull, are called *synarthroses.* A thin layer of fibrous connective tissue, called a *suture,* joins the bones of the joint together.

- ✓ **Slightly movable joints:** Joints that are slightly movable and connected by fibrocartilage or hyaline cartilage are called *amphiarthroses.* An example of this type of joint includes the *intervertebral disks,* which join each vertebra and allow slight movement of the vertebral column.

- ✓ **Freely movable joints:** Joints that are freely movable are called *diarthroses.* They're also called *synovial joints* because a cavity between the two connecting bones is lined with a synovial membrane and filled with *synovial fluid,* which helps to lubricate and cushion the joint. The ends of the bones are cushioned by hyaline cartilage. Diarthroses are joined together by ligaments. The following list shows the many types of diarthroses:

  - • **Ball-and-socket joints:** With this joint, the ball-shaped head of one bone fits into a depression (socket) in another bone. This joint, which can move in all planes, allows circular movements and rotation. Examples of this type of joint include the shoulder and the hip.

  - • **Condyloid joints:** With this joint, the oval-shaped condyle of one bone fits into the oval-shaped cavity of another bone. This joint can move in different planes but can't rotate. An example of this type of joint is the knuckles (the joints between the metacarpals and the phalanges).

  - • **Gliding joints:** This joint joins flat or slightly curved surfaces and allows sliding or twisting in different planes. Examples include the joints between the carpal bones (wrist) and between the tarsal bones (ankle).

  - • **Hinge joints:** With this joint, a convex surface joins with a concave surface. This joint provides up and down motion in one plane, so it either bends (flexes) or straightens (extends). Examples of this joint include elbows and knees.

- **Pivot joint:** With this joint, a cylinder-shaped projection on one bone is surrounded by a ring of another bone and ligament. Rotation is the only possible movement with this joint. Examples include the joint between the radius and ulna at the elbow and the joint atlas and axis at the top of the vertebral column.

- **Saddle joint:** With this joint, each bone is saddle shaped and fits into the saddle-shaped region of the opposite bone. Many movements are possible with this joint; it can move in different planes but it can't rotate. An example is the joint between the carpal and metacarpal bones of the thumb.

Discovering what your joints can do

Your joints perform either angular or circular movements. *Angular* movements make the angle formed by two bones larger or smaller. Examples of these movements include the following:

- ✔ **Abduction** moves a body part to the side, away from the body's middle. When you make a snow angel and move your arms and legs out and up, that's abduction.

- ✔ **Adduction** moves a body part from the side toward the body's middle. When you're in the snow angel position and you move your arms and legs back down, that's adduction.

- ✔ **Extension** makes the angle larger. *Hyperextension* occurs when the body part moves beyond a straight line (180 degrees).

- ✔ **Flexion** decreases the joint angle. When you flex your arm, for example, you move your forearm to your arm.

Circular movements occur only at ball-and-socket joints like in the hip or shoulder. Examples of circular movements include the following:

- ✔ **Circumduction** is the movement of a body part in circles.

- ✔ **Depression** is the downward movement of a body part.

- ✔ **Elevation** is the upward movement of a body part, such as shrugging your shoulders.

- ✔ **Eversion** only happens when the foot is turned so the sole is facing outward.

✔ **Inversion** only happens when the foot is turned so the sole is facing inward.

✔ **Rotation** is the movement of a body part around its own axis, such as shaking your head to answer "no."

✔ **Supination** and **pronation** refer to the arm, and they stem from the terms *supine* and *prone*. *Supination* is the rotation of the forearm to make the palm face upward or forward. *Pronation* is the rotation of the forearm to make the palm face downward or backward.

The 411 on the Muscular System

The human muscular system is always busy pulling things up, pushing things down and around, and moving things inside you and outside you. This section clues you in to the different jobs of your skeletal muscles, the various muscle tissue types, and the basics of muscle contraction.

Seeing what your skeletal muscles do

The *skeletal muscles,* the muscles that move your bones, comprise a substantial portion of your body mass, and most of what you eat goes to fuel their metabolism. In the following sections, you find out what they do with all that energy.

Support your structure

Muscles are attached to bones on the inside of your body and to skin on the outside, with various types of connective tissue between the layers. Thus, they hold your body together. Along with your skin and your skeleton, your muscles shield your internal organs from injury from impact or penetration.

As it does with everything else, gravity pulls your weight downward (toward the planet's center). But gravity doesn't only pull on the soles of your feet — it pulls on all your weight. If gravity had its way, you'd be lying on the floor right now. Thankfully, your muscles pull your weight up and hold you upright.

Move you

Contracting and releasing a muscle moves the bone it's attached to relative to the rest of the body. The movement of the bone, in turn, moves all the tissue attached to it, such as when you raise your arm. Certain combinations of these types of movements move the entire body, as when you walk, run, swim, skate, or dance.

Muscle contraction is responsible for little movements, too, like blinking your eyes, dilating your pupils, and smiling.

Position and balance you

A very close interaction outside of your conscious control between some muscle cells and the nervous system keeps you not just upright, but in balance. Nerve impulses throughout the muscular system cause muscles to contract or relax to oppose gravity in a more subtle way when, say, you're shifting your weight from one side to the other as you step. This interaction is called *muscle tone.*

When you step down a steep incline in rough terrain, your muscle tone brings your abs and your back muscles into action in a different way than when you step across your living room rug. The mechanisms of muscle tone may move your arms up and away from your body to counterbalance the pull of gravity with an accuracy and precision you could never calculate cognitively. Below your conscious level, the mechanisms of muscle tone are active every minute of every day, even when you're asleep.

Muscle tone relies on *muscle spindles,* which are specialized muscle cells that are wrapped with nerve fibers. The central nervous system stays in contact with the muscles through the muscle spindles. Spindles send messages about your body position through the spinal cord to the brain; to initiate the fine adjustments, the brain sends signals about which muscles to contract and which to release through the spinal cord and nerves to the muscle spindles.

Maintain your body temperature

Muscle contributes to *homeostasis* by generating heat to balance the loss of heat from the body surface. Muscle contraction uses energy from the breakdown of ATP and generates heat as a byproduct. The heat generated by the muscles interacts with other physiological processes that release heat from the body — sweating, for example — to maintain thermoregulation. Similarly, shivering is a series of muscle contractions that generate extra heat to increase your temperature in cold situations.

Push things around inside you

Following are some of the muscles that keep things moving within your body, all without any thought from you:

- **Cardiac muscle:** The heart is a muscle that contracts rhythmically, pumping blood into the arteries. A muscular lining in the arteries rhythmically dilates and contracts, pushing blood along with enough force (blood pressure) to drive this relatively viscous fluid into the capillary beds. The rhythmic movements of the heart and arteries are detectable as your pulse.

  The ability of the arterial wall muscles to dilate and contract in response to physiological stimuli enables the subtle control of blood pressure. Damage to this muscular lining causes *arteriosclerosis* (hardening of the arteries), which inhibits the muscle lining's ability to move (dilate and contract) the vessel, an underlying factor in cardiovascular disease and dysfunction.

- **Diaphragm:** The *diaphragm* is a skeletal muscle whose contraction and release forces air in and out of the lungs.

- **Digestive smooth muscle:** Your digestive system is lined with a kind of muscle tissue called *smooth muscle* that contracts in pulsating waves, pushing ingested material along the digestive tract. Think of this muscular lining as a conveyor belt on a disassembly line. Refer to Chapter 6 for details.

- **Sphincter muscles:** These muscles are essentially valves: rings of smooth muscle that are fully in contraction in their resting state, holding some material in one place, and then relaxing only briefly to allow the material to move through. You find sphincters at various places in the digestive system, from the very beginning to the very end, and in other parts of the body as well.

Taking a look at tissue types

A muscle tissue type isn't the same as a muscle. Your left bicep is a muscle; in all, you have hundreds of named muscles. However, you have only three muscle tissue types: *skeletal muscle tissue, cardiac muscle tissue,* and *smooth muscle tissue.* The following sections fill you in on each type as well as the cellular characteristics of muscle tissue.

Browsing the unique features of muscle cells

Your muscle tissue is made up of cells that are different from the other cells of your body. These cells are so unique that they're even different from each other based on the type of muscle tissue they belong to. The three muscle types are distinguishable anatomically by their characteristic cells and structures. They're also distinguishable physiologically as *voluntary* or *involuntary.*

Muscle cells feature these characteristics, which you can see in Figure 3-2:

- ✓ **Single or multiple nuclei:** Cardiac muscle cells and smooth muscle cells have one nucleus apiece, like most other cells. Skeletal muscle cells (fibers), however, are *multinucleate,* meaning they have numerous nuclei within one cell membrane.

  Skeletal muscle cells don't grow these extra nuclei; during the development of skeletal muscle tissue, numerous skeletal muscle cells merge into one large cell, and most of the nuclei are retained within one continuous cell membrane, along with most of the mitochondria. (For the scoop on mitochondria and other components of cells, see Chapter 2.)

- ✓ **Striation:** Skeletal muscle is *striated,* meaning that, under a microscope, alternating light and dark bands are visible in the muscle cell (fiber). Striation is the result of the subcellular structure of skeletal muscle cells (as explained in the later section "Reviewing skeletal muscle") and is integral to the mechanism of contraction called the *sliding filament model* (which we explain in the later section "Making muscles contract: The sliding filament model").

Cardiac muscle cells are striated as well, and they also contract by a variation of the sliding filament model. Smooth muscle cells aren't striated in appearance but do follow a version of the sliding filament model.

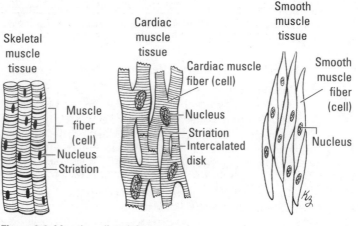

Figure 3-2: Muscle cell and tissue types.

Muscle cells can also be categorized by the type of contraction they perform. They can be categorized as one of the following:

✔ **Involuntary:** Smooth and cardiac muscle cells are *involuntary,* meaning their contraction is initiated and controlled by parts of the nervous system that are far from the conscious level of the brain. You have no practical way to consciously control, or even become aware of, the smooth muscle contractions in your stomach that are grinding up this morning's muffin.

✔ **Voluntary:** Skeletal muscle is classified as *voluntary* because you make a decision at the conscious level to move the muscle. For example, when you decide to reach for a doorknob and turn it, your muscles carry out the command from your brain to do so.

Table 3-2 sums up the characteristics and classifications of muscle cells.

Table 3-2   Cell Characteristics of Muscle Cells

	Skeletal	*Cardiac*	*Smooth*
Multinucleate	Yes	No	No
Striated	Yes	Yes	No
Voluntary	Yes	No	No

Reviewing skeletal muscle

Skeletal muscle tissue is made of bundles of fibers. Like fibrous material of every kind, skeletal muscle tissue gets its strength from assembling individual fibers together into strands, and then bundling and rebundling the strands. Two properties make this particular fibrous material special: The strands are made of protein, and they renew and repair themselves constantly. See Figure 3-3 for details of skeletal muscle tissue anatomy.

Homing in on the cellular level

Individual muscle cells, which physiologists call *fibers,* are slender cylinders that sometimes run the entire length of a muscle. Each fiber (cell) has many nuclei located along its length and close to the cell membrane, which is called the *sarcolemma.* Outside the sarcolemma is a lining called the *endomysium,* a type of connective tissue.

Muscle *spindles* are specialized skeletal muscle fibers that are wrapped with nerve fibers. Figure 3-3 shows how skeletal muscle is connected to the nervous system. Spindles are distributed throughout the muscle tissue and provide sensory information to the central nervous system.

Within the muscle fibers are *myofibrils.* The myofibrils are composed of *sarcomeres,* which are distinct units arranged linearly (end to end) along the length of the myofibril. Muscle contraction occurs within the sarcomere. (Refer to the later section "Making muscles contract: The sliding filament model" for more on muscle contraction within sarcomeres.)

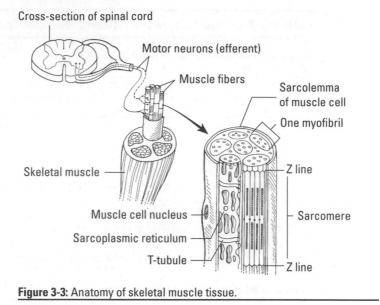

Cross-section of spinal cord

Motor neurons (efferent)

Muscle fibers

Sarcolemma of muscle cell

One myofibril

Skeletal muscle

Z line

Muscle cell nucleus

Sarcomere

Sarcoplasmic reticulum

T-tubule

Z line

Figure 3-3: Anatomy of skeletal muscle tissue.

Examining the tissue level

Muscle fibers are bound together into bundles called *fascicles*. Each fascicle is bound by a connective-tissue lining called a *perimysium*. Spindle fibers are distributed throughout each fascicle. The fascicles are then bound together to form a muscle, a discrete assembly of skeletal muscle tissue, with a connective-tissue wrapper called an *epimysium* holding the whole package together.

Tendons — ropy extensions of the connective tissue covering the skeletal bones — grow into the epimysium, holding the muscle firmly to the bone.

How many ways can you say "fiber"? Anatomists need them all when they're talking about the muscular system. Make sure you're thinking at the right level of organization (*subcellular, cellular,* or *tissue*) when you see these terms: *filament, myofibril, fiber,* and *fascicle.*

Working together: Synergists and antagonists

Groups of skeletal muscles that contract simultaneously to move a body part are said to be *synergistic.* The muscle that does most of the moving is the *prime mover.* The muscles that help the prime mover achieve a certain body movement are *synergists*. For example, when you move your elbow joint, the bicep is the prime mover and the brachioradialis stabilizes the joint, thus aiding the motion.

Antagonistic muscles also act together to move a body part, but one group contracts while the other releases in a kind of push-pull game. One example is flexing your arm. When you bend your forearm up toward your shoulder, your biceps muscle contracts, but the triceps muscle in the back of your arm relaxes. The actions of the biceps and triceps muscles are opposite, but you need both actions to allow you to flex your arm. Antagonistic actions lower your arm, too: The biceps relaxes, and the triceps contracts.

Checking out cardiac muscle

The heart has its own very special type of muscle tissue, called *cardiac muscle*. The cells (fibers) in cardiac muscle contain one nucleus (they're *uninucleated*) and are cylindrical; they may be branched in shape. Unlike skeletal muscle, where the fibers lie alongside one another, cardiac muscle fibers interlock, which promotes the rapid transmission of the contraction impulse throughout the heart. Cardiac muscle cells are striated, like skeletal muscle cells, and cardiac muscle contraction is involuntary, like smooth muscle contraction. Cardiac muscle fibers contract in a way similar to skeletal muscle fibers, by a sliding filament mechanism.

Cardiac muscle tissue is on the job, day and night, from before birth to the moment of death. Throughout your lifetime, the cardiac muscle cells contract regularly and simultaneously hundreds of millions of times. When cardiac muscle tissue gives up, the game is over.

Unlike skeletal muscle and smooth muscle, contraction of the heart muscle is *autonomous,* which means it occurs without stimulation by a nerve. In between contractions, the fibers relax completely.

Considering smooth muscle

Smooth muscle tissue lines the organs and structures of many organ systems, including the digestive system, the urinary system, the respiratory system, the circulatory system, and the reproductive system. Smooth muscle tissue is fundamentally different from skeletal muscle tissue and cardiac muscle tissue in terms of cell structure and physiological function. However, smooth muscle sarcomeres are similar, and contraction is affected by a variation of the sliding filament model.

Smooth muscle cells (fibers) are *fusiform* (thick in the middle and tapered at the ends) and arranged to form sheets of tissue. Smooth muscle cells aren't striated. However, smooth muscle contractions are affected by a similar sliding filament mechanism as skeletal muscle cells (see the following section for more).

Smooth muscle contraction is typically slow, strong, and enduring. Smooth muscle can hold a contraction longer than skeletal muscle. In fact, some smooth muscles, notably the sphincters, are in a constant or nearly constant state of contraction. Childbirth is among the few occasions in life when humans (some humans, anyway) consciously experience smooth muscle contraction (although they don't consciously control it).

Making muscles contract: The sliding filament model

A muscle contracts when all the sarcomeres in all the myofibrils in all the fibers (cells) contract all together. The *sarcomere* is the functional unit within the *myofibril*. (Sarcomeres line up end to end along the myofibril.) The *sliding filament model* describes the fine points of how this contraction happens.

The key to the sliding filament model is the distinctive shapes of the protein molecules *myosin* and *actin* and their partial overlap in the sarcomere. The special chemistry of ATP supplies the energy for the filaments' movement. The following sections explain how sarcomeres create muscle contraction.

Assembling a sarcomere

The sarcomere is composed of *thick filaments* and *thin filaments*. The thick filaments are molecules of the protein *myosin*, which is dense and rubbery. The thin filaments are primarily made up of two strands of the lighter (less dense) protein *actin*, wrapped in a double helix, which, as in DNA, is springy.

The thin and thick filaments line up together in an orderly way to form a sarcomere. One end of a thin filament touches and adjoins the end of another thin filament. Adjoined thin filaments adjust themselves so the joining points form a structure called a *Z line* — a straight line that runs perpendicular to the filament axis. The sarcomere begins at one Z line and ends at the next Z line. The thick filaments line up precisely between the thin filaments. Sarcomeres and Z lines are shown in Figure 3-3.

The two types of filaments overlap only partially when the sarcomere is at rest. The partial overlap gives skeletal muscle cells their *striations*. Where thick and thin filaments overlap, the tissue appears dark (dark band); where only thin filaments are present, the tissue appears lighter (light band).

Contracting and releasing the sarcomere

Myosin molecules have binding sites with a high affinity for ATP (refer to Chapter 1 for details on ATP). Actin molecules have binding sites with a high affinity for myosin. When a nerve impulse sends calcium ions into the cytoplasm of the muscle fiber, things start to happen.

The binding of calcium ions on actin molecules exposes the myosin binding sites of actin. Myosin, with its ATP cargo, binds to actin, forming cross-bridges between the thick and thin (actin) filaments of the sarcomere. The bond with actin distorts the myosin-ATP binding site, leading to the hydrolysis of the ATP and the release of its energy. This energy fuels the motion of the cross-bridges that pulls (slides) the thin filaments past the thick filaments toward the middle of the sarcomere. The distance between the Z lines becomes shorter because the length of the nonoverlapping portion of the two types of filaments becomes shorter. All sarcomeres in a fiber contract simultaneously, transmitting the force to the fiber ends.

The myosin then drops the products of the hydrolysis (ADP and P_i) from the binding site. Another molecule of ATP takes its place, reshaping the myosin molecule once again and pulling the actin-myosin bond apart. At this point, the cycle begins again.

Both the binding action and the release action require energy in the form of ATP. One molecule of ATP is needed for each binding and each release of each filament pair within each sarcomere. Thousands of molecules of ATP are required for every second of muscle contraction.

An Introduction to the Integument

The entity known as *you* is bounded by your integument. Everything inside the outermost layer of skin is *you*. Everything outside the outermost layer of skin is *not you*.

Your skin mediates much of the interaction between *you* and *not you*, which we henceforth call the *environment*. Your integument identifies *you* to other humans, a very important function for members of the hypersocial human species. Here's a look at the integument's other important functions:

✔ **Incoming messages:** Many types of sensory organs are embedded in your skin, including receptors for heat and cold, pressure, vibration, and pain.

✔ **Outgoing messages:** The skin and hair are messengers to the outside environment, mainly to other humans. People get information about your state of health (physical and emotional) by looking at your skin and hair. Your emotional state is signaled by pallor, flushing, blushing, goose bumps, sweating, and more. The odors of sweat from certain sweat glands signal sexual arousal.

✔ **Protection:** Skin protects the rest of the body by keeping out many threats from the environment, such as infection and predation by other organisms, damaging solar radiation, and nasty substances everywhere.

✔ **Substance production:** *Sebaceous glands* in the skin, usually associated with a hair follicle, produce a waxy substance called *sebum*. Similarly, sweat glands in the skin make sweat. In fact, your skin has several different types of glands, and each makes a specific type of sweat. Also, skin cells produce *keratin*, a fibrous protein that's an important structural and functional component of skin and is, essentially, the only component of hair and nails.

✔ **Thermoregulation:** The skin supports *thermoregulation* (the maintenance of optimum body temperature) in several ways — by producing sweat, for example.

✔ **Water balance:** The skin's outer layers are more or less impermeable to water, keeping water and salts at an optimum level inside the body and preventing excess fluid loss. A small amount of excess water and some bodily waste (urea) are eliminated through the skin.

Studying up on the structure of the integument

Your skin, itself a thin layer, is made up of many layers. This layering is visible to the unaided eye because each layer is different from the others and the transitions between layers appear to be relatively abrupt. We look at the three layers of the integument — the epidermis, the dermis, and the subcutaneous layer (hypodermis) — in the following sections.

When describing the integument, we use *up* and *above* to mean "toward the surface of the body," and *down* and *below* to mean "toward the center of the body." Sometimes, anatomists use the terms *superficial* and *deep* to mean the same things, respectively.

Touching the epidermis

The most familiar aspect of the integument is the *epidermis,* the outermost surface that you see on yourself and other people. The epidermis feels soft, slightly oily, elastic, resilient, and strong. In some places, the surface has a dense cluster of coarse hairs; in other spots, it has a lighter covering of light hairs; and in a few places, it has no hairs at all. The nails cover the tips of the fingers and toes.

The epidermis itself is made up of four to five different layers not visible to the unaided eye, from the *stratum corneum* at the top to the *stratum germinativum* (or *stratum basale*) at the bottom. All layers of the epidermis are composed of stratified squamous epithelial tissue, but the layers perform different functions. The epidermis has no blood supply; it's nourished by diffusion from the dermis layer below.

Stratum corneum: The thin, impervious cover

Think of the *stratum corneum,* the top layer, as a sheet of self-repairing fiberglass over the other layers of the epidermis. It's only 25 to 30 cells thick, but it's dense and relatively hard. All the cells are *keratinocytes,* which produce the fibrous protein *keratin.*

The keratinocytes of the stratus corneum originate as squamous epithelial cells in the *stratum germinativum* (the bottom layer of the skin).

The uppermost surface of the stratum corneum is covered with a waxy, waterproof coating of *sebum*. This layer of the skin protects the entire body by making sure some things stay in and everything else stays out.

The stratum corneum doesn't seal out ultraviolet radiation. This form of energy goes directly through the skin's surface and down to the layers below, where it stimulates the production of vitamin D. In high doses, it burns the skin and damages DNA, which can cause cells to become cancerous. Evolution's response to the threat of UV-induced cell damage is the pigment *melanin*, which absorbs harmful UV-radiation and transforms the energy into harmless heat.

Stratum lucidum: The layer on the hands and feet

The *stratum lucidum*, found only on the palms of the hands and soles of the feet (thick skin), the *stratum granulosum*, and the *stratum spinosum* lie in distinct layers below the stratum corneum. Old cells slough off above and new cells push up from below, finally getting up into the stratum corneum. The process takes about 14 to 30 days. Like other epidermal cells, these cells live in the stratum corneum for about a month.

The keratinocytes produce *lipids* (fatty substances) and undergo successive stages of keratinization and other kinds of differentiation in these layers. These layers also contain *Langerhans cells*, immune system cells that arrest microbial invaders and transport them to the lymph nodes for destruction.

Stratum germinativum: The constantly renewing layer

The *stratum germinativum*, also called the *stratum basale* or *basal layer*, is like a cell farm, constantly producing new cells and pushing them up into the layer above. This stratum contains *melanocytes*, which produce the *melanin* pigment that gives color to your skin, hair, and eyes and protects the skin from the damaging effects of UV radiation in sunlight. Melanin absorbs UV radiation and dissipates more than 99.9 percent of it as heat.

Exploring the dermis

Below the layers of the epidermis (and several times thicker) is the *dermis*. The dermis itself is made up of two layers:

✔ **The papillary region:** This region consists of the *basement membrane*, which sits just below the epidermis, and the *papillae* (finger-like projections) that push into the basement membrane, increasing the area of contact between the dermis and the epidermis.

In your palms, fingers, soles, and toes, the papillae projecting into the epidermis form *friction ridges*. (They help your hand or foot to grasp by increasing friction.) The pattern of the friction ridges on a finger is called a *fingerprint*.

✔ **The reticular region:** This region is chock-full of protein fibers and is a complex and metabolically active layer. Cells (which migrate down from the epidermis during development) and structures of the reticular region manufacture many of the skin's characteristic products: hair and nails, sebum, and sweat. The region also contains structures that connect the integument to other organ systems: sensors of pressure (touch) and heat, lymph vessels, and a rich blood supply.

The blood vessels in the dermis provide nourishment and waste removal from the dermis's own cells as well as from the stratum germinativum. These blood vessels dilate when the body needs to lose heat and constrict to keep heat in. They also dilate and contract in response to your emotional state, brightening or darkening your skin color, thereby functioning as social signaling.

The sensory receptors in the dermis transmit sensations, such as pressure, vibration, and light touch, to the nervous system. The receptors are sprinkled throughout the dermis and are connected to the nerves that run through the dermis and subcutaneous layer. Not every inch of skin is covered with receptors for every sensation. So at one spot on your skin, you may sense light touch, while a few centimeters away, you may sense pressure.

Getting way under your skin: The subcutaneous layer

The *subcutaneous layer* (also known as the *hypodermis,* or *superficial fascia*) is the layer of tissue directly underneath the dermis. It's mainly composed of connective and *adipose* (fatty) tissue. Its physiological functions include insulation, the storage of energy, and help in the anchoring of the skin. The subcutaneous layer contains larger blood vessels, lymph vessels, and nerve fibers than those found in the dermis. Its loosely arranged elastin fibers anchor the hypodermis to the muscle below it.

The thickness of the subcutaneous layer is determined in some places by the amount of fat deposited into the cells of the adipose tissue, which makes up the majority of the subcutaneous layer.

Accessorizing your skin

This section has nothing to do with tattoos or body piercing. It's all about the *accessory structures* that work with your skin: hair, nails, and glands.

Locks, beards, and other hair

Your body has millions of hair follicles, about the same number as the chimpanzee, humanity's closest evolutionary relative. Like chimps, humans have hairless palms, soles, lips, and nipples. Unlike a chimpanzee, however, most of your hair is lightweight, fine, and downy. The hair on your head is coarser and longer to help hold in body heat. Puberty brings about a surge of sex hormones that stimulate hair growth in the *axillary* (armpit) and pelvic regions and, in males, on the face and neck.

A hair arises in a *hair follicle,* a small tube made of epidermal cells that extend down into the dermis to take advantage of its rich blood supply. Cells at the bottom of the hair follicle continually divide to produce new cells that are added to the end of the hair and push the older cells up through the layers of the epidermis. On their way up and out, the hair cells become keratinized.

Nails and nail beds

Your fingernails and toenails lie on a *nail bed.* At the back of the nail bed is the *nail root.* Just like skin and hair, nails start growing near the blood supply that lies under the nail bed, and the cells move outward at the rate of about 1 millimeter per week. As they move out over the nail bed, they become keratinized. At the bottom of your nails is a white, half-moon-shaped area called the *lunula.* (*Lun-* is the Latin root for moon, as in *lunar.*) The lunula is white because it's the area of cell growth. In the nail body, the nail appears pink because the blood vessels lie underneath the nail bed. But many more cells fill in the area of growth. This layer is thicker, and you see white instead of pink.

Glands

Glands in the skin make and secrete substances that are transported to your body's outer surface. The contraction of tiny muscles in the gland accomplishes this secretion. The two main types of skin glands are *sudoriferous glands* (sweat glands) and *sebaceous glands* (oil glands). Here's a rundown of each:

- ✓ **Sudoriferous glands:** Your body contains two types of sudoriferous glands:

  - *Eccrine sweat glands,* which are distributed all over the skin. These glands open to the skin's surface, and when you're hot, they let heat escape in the form of sweat to reduce body temperature by a process of evaporative cooling.

  - *Apocrine sweat glands,* which start to develop during puberty deep in the hair follicles of the armpits and groin. Apocrine sweat contains a milky white substance and may also contain *pheromones,* chemicals that communicate information to other individuals by altering their hormonal balance. Apocrine glands become active when you're anxious and stressed as well as when you're sexually stimulated. Bacteria on the skin that digest the milky white substance produce unpleasantly odiferous byproducts.

- ✓ **Sebaceous glands:** These glands secrete an oily substance called *sebum* into hair roots. Sebum helps maintain your hair in a healthy state, which is important in regulating body temperature. It flows out along the hair shaft, coating the hair and the epidermis, forming a protective, waterproof layer. Sebum prevents water loss to the outside. It also helps protect you from infection by making the skin surface an inhospitable place for some bacteria.

  In the watery environment of the amniotic sac, the human fetus produces a thick layer of sebum, called the *vernix caseosa.* Ear wax (*cerumen*) is a type of sebum produced by specialized cells in the ear canal.

Chapter 4

Getting to the Heart of the Circulatory System

●●●

In This Chapter

▶ Breaking down the heart's parts

▶ Discovering arteries, capillaries, and veins

▶ Uncovering blood's main components

▶ Following blood along its path through your body

●●●

*T*he circulatory system's main components are the heart and blood vessels. As a result, the functions of this system are all related to transportation. Nearly every substance made or used in the body is transported in the blood: hormones, gases of respiration, products of digestion, metabolic wastes, and immune system cells.

The blood also transports heat. Stimulated by the hormones of thermoregulation, blood flow can disperse heat to the environment at the body surface or conserve heat for essential functions in the body core.

In this chapter, we tell you what you need to know about the structures of your circulatory system and the blood it moves throughout your body. We also describe just how your circulatory system accomplishes its important task.

Analyzing the Cardiac Anatomy

The circulatory system — or *cardiovascular system* — consists of the heart and the blood vessels. The heart's pumping action (or beat) squeezes blood out of the heart, and the pressure it generates forces the blood through the blood vessels. The autonomic nervous system controls the rate of the heartbeat.

In this section, we provide a brief overview of the heart, including its shape and collection of tissues. We also explain how the heart uses veins and arteries to pump blood.

Examining the shape of the heart

The heart is shaped like a cone and is only about the size of your fist (see Figure 4-1). It lies between your lungs, just. behind your sternum, and the tip of the cone points to the left. In most individuals, the heart is situated slightly to the left of center in the chest.

The heart has four hollow spaces called *chambers*. The contraction of the heart muscle pumps blood into and out of all four chambers in a rhythmic pattern. (The arrows in Figure 4-2 show the direction of blood flow through the chambers.)

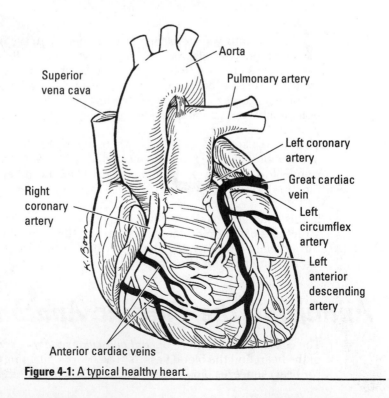

Figure 4-1: A typical healthy heart.

The heart is also divided anatomically and functionally into left and right sides. Each side of the heart has one *atrium* and one *ventricle,* each with a separate function. A membrane called the *interatrial septum* separates the atria; a membrane called the *interventricular septum* separates the ventricles.

Between the chambers are several *valves* that allow measured quantities of blood to flow into the chambers and keep blood flowing in the right direction. The valves' names tell you either their anatomical location or their characteristics. Consider the following:

- ✔ The two *atrioventricular* (AV) *valves* lie between the atrium and the ventricle on each side.

- ✔ The *bicuspid valve* (BV) has two flaps.

- ✔ The *tricuspid valve* (TV) has three flaps.

- ✔ The *semilunar valves* (SV) are shaped like half-moons.

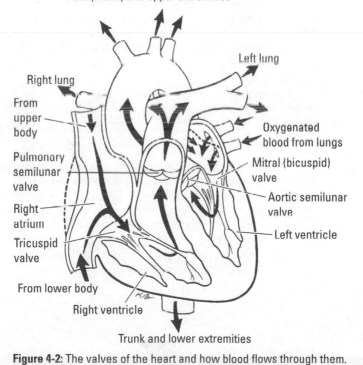

Figure 4-2: The valves of the heart and how blood flows through them.

Looking at the heart's tissues

The tissues of the heart perform the functions required to keep the double-pump working strongly and steadily. Like other hollow organs, the heart is made up of layers of endothelial and connective tissue. Here's the lowdown on those layers:

✔ **Endocardium:** The *endocardium* is a layer of endothelial tissue that lines the inside of the chambers. This layer is continuous with the vascular endothelium, which we talk about in detail in the later section "Beginning at the arteries."

✔ **Myocardium:** The *myocardium* (literally, "heart muscle") is the thick, muscular layer of your heart. It's composed of cardiac muscle fibers that contract in a coordinated way to pump the blood out of the heart and into the aorta with enough force to carry it through the arterial system and out into the capillaries.

✔ **Epicardium:** The *epicardium* is the visceral layer of the *serous pericardium* — a double layered sac that covers the heart. The epicardium is a conical sac of fibrous tissue that closely envelops the myocardium and surrounds the roots of the major blood vessels. It secretes *pericardial fluid* into the *pericardial cavity,* which lubricates the tissues as the heart beats.

✔ **Pericardial cavity:** The *pericardial cavity* is a fluid-filled space between the epicardium and the parietal layer of the serous pericardium. The fluid reduces friction between the pericardial membranes.

✔ **Parietal layer of the serous pericardium:** This layer is a serous membrane that's attached to the outermost layer of the heart, the *fibrous pericardium.* The fibrous pericardium is a thick, white sheet of fibrous connective tissue that anchors the heart and the major blood vessels, including the aorta, to the sternum and diaphragm. The parietal layer of the serous pericardium also secretes pericardial fluid into the pericardial cavity.

Observing how blood flows to (and from) the heart

Blood flows in and out of the heart every second of your life, and some of that blood needs to supply the cells of the heart itself with oxygen and nutrients. The coronary arteries supply oxygenated blood to the heart, while cardiac veins return deoxygenated blood to the pulmonary circulation loop. Here's some more info on each of these:

✔ **Coronary arteries:** Two large coronary arteries and their many branches supply blood to the heart. Large arteries enter the heart on the left and right at the top. They're called the left and right coronary arteries because they sit atop and encircle the heart, looking like a crown (see Figure 4-3).

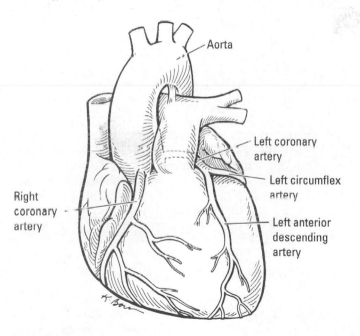

Figure 4-3: The coronary arteries.

The right coronary artery and its two major branches, the *marginal artery* and the *posterior interventricular artery,* primarily supply the right atrium and ventricle with oxygenated blood and nutrients. The left coronary artery and its two branches, the *anterior interventricular artery* and the *left circumflex coronary artery,* primarily supply the left atrium and ventricle with oxygenated blood and nutrients.

✔ **Cardiac veins:** The cardiac venous system is similarly branched, often lying alongside the coronary arteries and their branches. Like everything about the heart, the cardiac venous system is composed of two parts, left and right. The *left cardiac venous system,* also called the *coronary sinus system,* receives deoxygenated blood from most of the superficial veins of the heart. The *right cardiac venous system* is composed of veins that originate on the anterior and lateral surfaces of the right ventricle and drain directly into the right atrium. The smallest vessels (the *venae cordis minimae*) drain the myocardium directly into the atria and ventricles.

Meet Your Blood Vessels

Your blood vessels comprise a network of channels through which your blood flows. But the vessels aren't passive tubes. Rather, they're active organs that, when functioning properly, assist the heart in circulating the blood and influence the blood's constitution. The innermost layer of the heart and of all vessels is continuous — it's one convoluted sheet of epithelium.

The vessels that take blood away from the heart are *arteries.* The vessels that bring blood toward the heart are *veins.* (The smallest vessels are called *arterioles* and *venules,* respectively.) Generally, arteries have veins of the same size running right alongside or near them, and they often have similar names.

The arterial vessels (arteries and arterioles) decrease in diameter as they spread throughout the body. Eventually, they end in the *capillaries,* the tiny vessels that connect the arterial and venous systems. The venous vessels become increasingly larger as they converge on the heart. The smaller venules carry deoxygenated blood from a capillary to a vein, and the larger veins carry the deoxygenated blood from the venules back to the heart.

The following sections take a closer look at the three types of blood vessels.

Beginning at the arteries

Your arteries form a branching network of vessels, with the main trunk, called the *aorta,* arising from the left ventricle and splitting immediately into the *brachiocephalic trunk, left common carotid artery,* and *left subclavian artery,* which serve the head and upper limbs. The *descending aorta* — which serves the thoracic organs, abdominal organs, and lower limbs — gives off several branches:

- ✔ The *mesenteric arteries,* the main arteries of the digestive tract

- ✔ Two *renal arteries,* which supply the kidneys

- ✔ The *common iliac arteries,* which supply the pelvis and lower limbs

Although an artery looks like a simple tube, the anatomy is complex. As you can see in Figure 4-4, arteries are made of three concentric layers of tissue around a space, called the *lumen,* where the blood flows.

- ✔ **Tunica externa:** The outside layer, the *tunica externa,* is a thick layer of connective tissue that supports the vessel and protects the inner layers from harm. The larger the artery, the thicker the connective tissue supporting it. (However, this type of tissue can become stiff with age.)

- ✔ **Tunica media:** The next layer in, the *tunica media,* is a thick wall of smooth muscle and elastic tissue. This layer expands and contracts with every pulse wave (heartbeat), and sometimes it gives a little squeeze to increase the pressure and force the blood through.

- ✔ **Tunica intima:** The inner layer, the *tunica intima,* is a single-cell-thick endothelial layer that lines the lumen and is continuous through all the organs of the circulatory system. The *vascular endothelium,* as this tissue is also called, is active metabolically, releasing into the blood various substances that influence blood circulation and vascular health. It also specializes in transporting oxygen, nutrients, and other substances from the blood flowing in the lumen to the smooth muscle fibers of the tunica media.

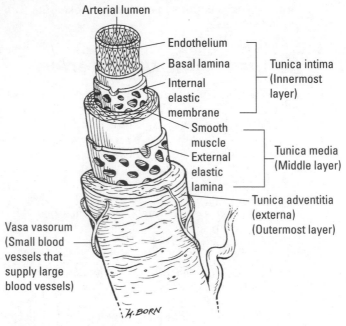

Arterial lumen

Endothelium ⎤
Basal lamina ⎟ Tunica intima
Internal ⎟ (Innermost
elastic ⎟ layer)
membrane ⎦

Smooth ⎤
muscle ⎟
External ⎟ Tunica media
elastic ⎟ (Middle layer)
lamina ⎦

Tunica adventitia
(externa)
(Outermost layer)

Vasa vasorum
(Small blood
vessels that
supply large
blood vessels)

H. BORN

Figure 4-4: The anatomy of an artery.

Moving on to the capillaries

After passing from the arteries and the arterioles, blood enters the capillaries, which lie between larger blood vessels in *capillary beds.* A capillary bed forms a bridge between the arterioles and the venules. Capillary beds are everywhere in your body, which is why you bleed anywhere that you even slightly cut your skin.

Your capillaries are your smallest vessels. Only the single-cell-thick epithelial layer surrounds the lumen. The *precapillary sphincters* of the *metarterioles* can tighten or relax to control blood flow into the capillary bed.

Lacking the structure and complexity of arteries and veins, capillaries rely on simple diffusion to do their job, which consists of moving oxygen and nutrients from the blood to the cells and waste materials from the cells to the blood. *Capillary exchange* is the term used to describe these processes (see Figure 4-5).

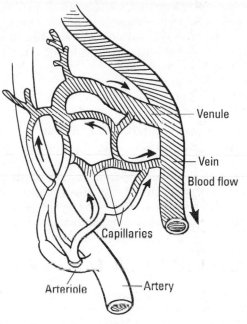

Figure 4-5: Capillary exchange.

The capillaries come into close contact with all the cells of your tissues. Consider the diffusion that occurs at both ends:

- **At the end near the arteriole,** oxygen diffuses out of the red blood cells and nutrient molecules diffuse out of the plasma, across the capillary membrane, and directly into the tissue fluid. The oxygen and nutrients dissolved in the tissue fluid diffuse across the membrane of the adjacent cells.

- **At the venule end,** the carbon dioxide and other waste materials diffuse out of the tissue fluid and across the capillary membrane into the blood. Then, the blood continues on through the venous system, and those waste materials are deposited in the proper locations on their way out of the body. The carbon dioxide diffuses out of the bloodstream in the lungs so it can be exhaled and thus removed from the body; other metabolic waste is filtered through the kidneys.

Besides aiding in the exchange of gases and nutrients throughout your body, capillaries serve two other important functions:

✔ **Thermoregulation:** Precapillary sphincters tighten when you're in a cold environment to prevent heat loss from the blood at the skin surface. Blood is then shunted from an arteriole directly to a venule through a nearby *arteriovenous shunt.* When you're in a warm environment or you're producing heat through exertion, the precapillary sphincters relax, opening the capillary bed to blood flow and dispersing heat.

✔ **Blood pressure regulation:** When blood pressure (blood volume) is low, the hormones that regulate this pressure stimulate the precapillary sphincters to tighten, temporarily reducing the total volume of the blood vessel system and thus raising the pressure. When blood pressure is high, they stimulate the sphincters to relax, increasing overall system volume and reducing pressure.

Traveling through the veins

Small veins converge into larger veins, all merging in the *inferior vena cava* and *superior vena cava,* the largest vessels in the venous system. These major veins return blood from below and above the heart, respectively. The inferior vena cava lies to the right of, and more or less parallel to, the descending aorta. The superior vena cava lies to the right of, and more or less parallel to, the aorta.

Veins have a similar anatomy to arteries, but they tend to be wider and their walls thinner and less elastic. The tunica interna of a vein is also part of the continuous endothelial layer that lines the whole network. The tunica media has a layer of elastic tissue and smooth muscle, but this layer is much thinner in a vein than in an artery. The veins have virtually no blood pressure, so they don't need a thick muscle layer to vary the vessel diameter or withstand fluid pressure. The outermost tunica externa is the thickest layer of a vein.

Because veins don't have a thick muscle layer to push blood through them, they depend on contraction of skeletal muscles to move blood back to the heart. As you move your arms, legs, and torso, your muscles contract, and those movements massage the blood through your veins. The blood moves through the vein a little bit at a time. The larger veins have valves that keep blood from flowing backward. The valves open in the direction that the blood is moving and then shut after the blood passes through to keep the blood heading toward the heart.

Here are the details on how veins work in each of the different parts of the body:

- **In the lower body:** The *internal iliac veins,* which return blood from the pelvic organs, and the *external iliac veins,* which return blood from the lower extremities, converge into the *common iliac veins.* The *renal veins* return blood from the kidneys. Both of these major veins flow into the inferior vena cava.

- **In the digestive tract:** Blood from the digestive tract travels in the *hepatic portal vein* to the liver (see Figure 4-6). Specialized cells in the liver move glucose molecules from the blood into storage. Phagocytic cells in the liver destroy bacterial cells that make it through the digestive process and remove toxins and other foreign material from the blood. Blood exits the liver through the *hepatic veins,* which flow into the inferior vena cava. The inferior vena cava empties into the right atrium.

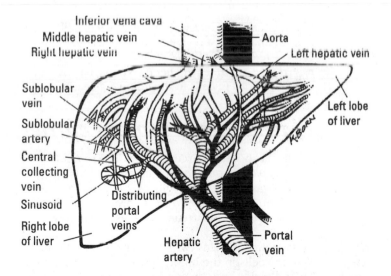

Figure 4-6: Hepatic portal system (venous circulation).

✔ **In the head and upper extremities:** Deoxygenated blood from the head and upper extremities drains into the *brachiocephalic veins.* The veins of the upper extremity — the *ulnar veins, radial veins,* and *subclavian veins* — also drain into the brachiocephalic veins. The *jugular veins* of the head and neck also drain into the brachiocephalic veins, which connect to the superior vena cava, which enters the right atrium.

After the blood from the right atrium has been pumped into the right ventricle, it's pumped into the lungs, where the blood is oxygenated, and then it flows back to the heart in the *pulmonary veins,* the only veins that carry oxygenated (red) blood.

Discovering What's in Your Blood

Blood — that deep maroon, body-temperature-warm liquid that courses through your body — is a vitally important, life-supporting, life-giving, life-saving substance that everybody needs. And every adult-size body contains about 5 quarts of the precious stuff.

Blood consists of many different types of cells in a matrix called *plasma,* making it a connective tissue. The different types of cells — *red blood cells, white blood cells,* and *platelets* — are referred to as *formed elements.* We discuss plasma and these different types of cells in the following sections.

Plasma: Your protein carrier

Plasma is about 92 percent water. The remaining 8 percent is made of *plasma proteins,* including salt ions, oxygen and carbon dioxide gases, nutrients (glucose, fats, amino acids) from the foods you take in, *urea* (a waste product), and other substances carried in the bloodstream, such as hormones and enzymes.

The plasma proteins, which are produced in the liver or by immune cells in the blood, have some important functions. The following are some example of plasma proteins:

✓ **Albumin:** The smallest plasma protein and the most abundant, albumin maintains the *osmotic pressure* in the bloodstream within the homeostatic range.

✓ **Fibrinogen:** During the process of clot formation, fibrinogen is converted into threads of *fibrin,* which form a meshlike structure that traps blood cells to form a clot.

✓ **Immunoglobulin (antibody):** These proteins are created in response to an invading microbe by cells that make up the immune system (turn to Chapter 9 for more on the immune system).

Red blood cells: In charge of moving O_2 and CO_2

Red blood cells (RBCs), or *erythrocytes* (*erythro* is the Greek word for "red"), are the most numerous of the blood cells and one of the most numerous of all cell types in your body. About one-quarter of the body's approximately 3 trillion cells are RBCs. They're among the cell types that must be constantly regenerated and disposed of. In fact, you produce and destroy a few million RBCs every second!

The cytoplasm of RBCs is full to the brim with an iron-containing biomolecule called *hemoglobin.* The iron-containing heme group in hemoglobin binds oxygen at the respiratory membrane and then releases it in the capillaries. The ability of hemoglobin to bind and release oxygen is the sole mechanism by which all your cells and tissues get the oxygen they need to sustain their metabolism. RBCs containing heme-bound oxygen are bright red, the familiar color of the arterial blood that flows from wounds. RBCs in the venous system have less heme-bound oxygen and are a dark red.

As oxygen diffuses into a cell, carbon dioxide diffuses out, making its way in the interstitial fluid to the venous system. Some deoxygenated hemoglobin in the venous blood takes up carbon dioxide to form *carboxyhemoglobin.* At the respiratory membrane, carboxyhemoglobin releases the carbon dioxide and takes up oxygen again. Carbon dioxide is transported in several different ways in the blood to the respiratory membrane, where it enters the lung and is exhaled in the breath.

An RBC has about a four-month life span, at the end of which it's destroyed by a *phagocyte* (a large cell with cleanup responsibilities) in the liver or spleen. The iron is removed from the heme group and is transferred to either the liver (for storage) or the bone marrow (for use in the production of new hemoglobin). The rest of the heme group is converted to *bilirubin* and released into the plasma (giving plasma its characteristic straw color). The liver uses the bilirubin to form bile to help with the digestion of fats.

Platelets: The clotting cells

Platelets are tiny pieces of cells. Large cells in the red bone marrow called *megakaryocytes* break into fragments, which are the platelets. Their job is to begin the clotting process and plug up injured blood vessels. Platelets, also called *thrombocytes* (*thrombos* means "clot"), have a short life span — they live only about ten days.

White blood cells: The body's defenders

White blood cells (WBCs), also known as your immune cells, are derived from the same type of hematopoietic stem cells as RBCs. However, they take different paths early in the process of differentiation. The WBCs, also called *leukocytes* (except for the T-lymphocytes), leave the red bone marrow and enter into circulation in their mature form.

Focusing on the Physiology of Circulation

Your body makes it happen 100,000 times every day. Waking or sleeping, from a moment early in fetal development until the moment you die, the beat goes on. It may speed up slightly when you're working hard physically or you're excited or stressed, and some people can slow theirs down with meditation techniques. But for most people, it just plugs along, the same thing over and over.

What are we talking about? The heartbeat, of course. Your beating heart pushes blood around a double-circuit — out through your arteries, ultimately into your capillary beds, across your capillary beds and into your veins, and then back through your veins. The blood passes through the heart to the lungs and then back to the heart and out through the arteries again. Each complete double-circuit takes less than one minute.

You can feel the rhythmic pulsation of blood flow at certain spots around your body, most commonly on the inside of the wrist or on the carotid artery of the neck. What you feel as you touch these spots is your artery expanding as the blood rushes through it and then immediately returning to its normal size when the bulge of blood has passed.

The cardiac cycle: Conducting electricity

Five structures of the heart, together called the *cardiac conduction system*, specialize in initiating and conducting the electrical impulses that induce your heartbeat, keeping it regular and strong in every part of the organ (see Figure 4-7). We tell you about each structure and walk you through the cardiac cycle in the following sections.

Anatomy of cardiac conduction

The cardiac conduction system is made up of the following five structures:

- ✔ **Sinoatrial node (SA node; also called the sinus node):** A small knot of cardiac musclelike tissue (the pacemaker cells look like cardiac muscle cells, but they've lost the ability to contract) located on the back wall of the right atrium, near where the superior vena cava enters the heart. The SA node's cells initiate the electrical impulses that generate the heartbeat.

- ✔ **Atrioventricular node (AV node):** A small mass of tissue located in the right atrium near the septum that divides the right and left atria from the ventricles. Its function is to relay the impulses it receives from the SA node to the next part of the conduction system.

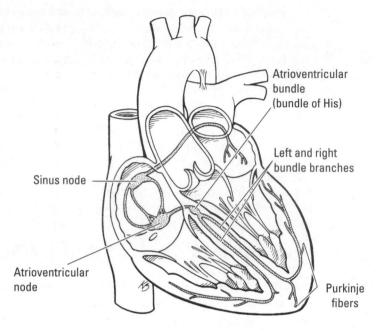

Figure 4-7: The conduction system of the heart.

✔ **Atrioventricular bundle (AV bundle):** A bundle of fibers that extends from the AV node into the *interventricular septum* (which divides the heart into right and left sides). The AV bundle transmits cardiac impulses.

✔ **Left and right bundle branches:** Where the septum widens, the AV bundle splits into the right and left bundle branches, each extending down under the endocardium and up along the outside of the ventricles. These bundles carry cardiac impulses.

✔ **Purkinje fibers:** At the ends of the AV bundle branches are the Purkinje fibers, which deliver impulses to the myocardial cells, causing the ventricles to contract.

The sequence of events

The cardiac conduction system is responsible for keeping the cardiac cycle going. If the cardiac cycle stops for too long, you experience serious consequences. Here's how the cycle goes:

1. **The electrical impulse is initiated in the SA node.** The right and left atria contract simultaneously, pumping blood into the right and left ventricles, respectively.

2. **The impulse passes to the AV node, which sends it to the AV bundle.** In the meantime, the right and left atria relax.

3. **The impulse passes into the right and left bundle branches and ultimately into the Purkinje fibers, causing the right ventricle to contract and pump its deoxygenated blood into the pulmonary arteries and lungs.** Simultaneously, the left ventricle contracts, pumping oxygenated blood into the aorta.

4. **The ventricles relax while the atria begin contracting, and the cycle starts all over again.**

Problems with signal conduction due to disease or abnormalities of the conducting system can occur anywhere along the heart's conduction pathway. Abnormally conducted signals resulting in irregular heartbeat are called *arrhythmias* or *dysrhythmias*.

On the beating path: Blood flow through the heart and body

The heart is a double-pump, so it has two circuits:

✔ **Pulmonary circulation:** This path goes from the heart to the lungs and back to the heart.

✔ **Systemic circulation:** This path goes from the heart to the body and back to the heart.

Every drop of your blood travels around this double-circuit about once per minute. You can see both paths in Figure 4-8.

Pulmonary circulation

Deoxygenated blood enters the heart's right atrium from the largest veins in the body, the superior vena cava and the inferior vena cava. When the SA node initiates the cardiac conduction cycle, the right atrium contracts and pumps the blood into the right ventricle.

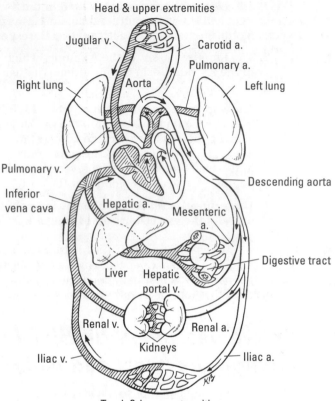

Head & upper extremities

Jugular v.

Carotid a.

Pulmonary a.

Right lung

Aorta

Left lung

Pulmonary v.

Descending aorta

Inferior vena cava

Hepatic a.

Mesenteric a.

Digestive tract

Liver Hepatic portal v.

Renal v.

Renal a.

Kidneys

Iliac v.

Iliac a.

Trunk & lower extremities

Figure 4-8: Pulmonary and systemic circulation working together through arterial and venous systems.

When the impulse passes to the AV node and then on to the AV bundle, the right bundle branch, and the Purkinje fibers, the right ventricle contracts, pumping blood into the pulmonary arteries, which take it to the lungs for gas exchange. During the relaxation phase of the atria, the newly oxygenated blood flows into the left atrium.

The pulmonary arteries are the only arteries that carry deoxygenated blood.

Systemic circulation

When the SA node initiates the cardiac conduction cycle, the left atrium contracts, pumping the oxygenated blood into the left ventricle.

When the impulse passes to the AV node and on to the AV bundle, the left bundle branch, and the Purkinje fibers, the left ventricle contracts and pumps blood into the aorta. From the aorta, the blood travels through the arteries and arterioles to the capillary beds and then back to the heart through the veins. During the relaxation phase of the atria, the deoxygenated blood flows into the right atrium.

Measuring the importance of blood pressure

Blood pressure is a term used to describe the force of blood pushing against the wall of an artery. It's measured in millimeters of mercury at both the highest point (*systole,* when the heart is contracted) and the lowest point (*diastole,* when the heart is relaxed) in the cardiac cycle. The systole pressure is always higher than the diastole. The higher the systolic and diastolic values, the more pressure present on the walls of the arteries. Two factors affect the blood pressure:

- ✔ **Cardiac output:** The amount of blood the heart pumps out per unit of time

- ✔ **Peripheral resistance:** A measure of the diameter and elasticity of the vessel walls

The cardiac output is determined by the heartbeat rate and the blood volume put out from a ventricle during one beat. When either of these rises, the blood pressure rises. Heart rate is increased by physical exertion, the release of epinephrine (a hormone), and other factors. The blood volume is influenced by the action of ADH (antidiuretic hormone) and other mechanisms in the kidneys to control the amount of water that's removed from the urine and restored to the blood.

The arteries' diameter changes locally and continuously. The pressure of the pulse wave increases pressure on the vascular endothelium, inducing it to release molecules, mainly nitrous oxide, that induce relaxation in the tunica media. The endothelium's ability to respond to the pulse-wave pressure is extremely important to vascular health. Resistance in the arteries to expansion as the blood rushes through raises the blood pressure.

As part of homeostasis, receptors in the arteries called *pressoreceptors* measure blood pressure. If the blood pressure is above the normal range, the brain sends out impulses to cause responses that decrease the heart rate and dilate the arterioles, both of which decrease blood pressure.

Hemostasis: Stopping the flow

Not the least amazing thing about blood is its ability to stop flowing. The term for this is *hemostasis* (literally, "blood stopping"), which is not to be confused with *homeostasis*.

Hemostasis is the reason you didn't bleed to death the first time you cut yourself. When vessels are cut, blood flows only long enough to clean the cut. As you watch, the blood stops flowing, and a plug, called a *clot,* forms. Within a day or so, the clot has dried and hardened into a scaly scab. Eventually, the scab falls off, revealing fresh new skin.

A blood clot consists of a plug of platelets enmeshed in a network of insoluble fibrin molecules. The *clotting cascade* is a physiological pathway that involves numerous components in the blood itself interacting to create a barrier to the flow. As soon as a blood vessel is injured, a signal is sent from the vascular endothelium to the platelets, summoning them to the injury site. On exposure to the air, their membranes become sticky, and they start to adhere together. Proteins in the blood plasma, called *coagulation factors* or *clotting factors,* respond in a complex cascade to form fibrin strands, which strengthen the platelet plug. Within minutes, your blood is safe in your body, where it belongs.

A blood clot in the right place is something to be grateful for. But blood tends to start clotting whenever it's not flowing freely, and this tendency can cause problems in the peripheral vessels (the arteries and veins of the legs). Clots also form on the inner wall of blood vessels when the endothelium is injured by disturbances in blood flow (turbulence) or by free radicals in the blood. These tiny clots adhere to the wall, further disturbing flow and causing more turbulence and more injury. Atherosclerotic plaque may begin to form around the clot. Worst of all, perhaps, is when the clot, with the plaque attached, breaks off from the vessel wall and floats free (sort of) in the bloodstream. Sooner or later, this *embolus* lodges somewhere in a vessel, sometimes with sudden and fatal consequences.

Chapter 5

Taking a Deep Breath with the Respiratory System

*V*ertebrates evolved in the sea from animals that obtained their oxygen by breathing water. Whatever it was that drove a fish to leave the watery environment, the challenge of breathing the gaseous atmosphere instead had to be met. All the major groups of land vertebrates (amphibians, reptiles, birds, and mammals) have succeeded by evolving the anatomy and physiology for breathing air. That anatomy and physiology makes up the respiratory system, which we discuss in this chapter.

Surveying the Duties of the Respiratory System

Air is the source of the oxygen your cells need for nearly all reactions. Your respiratory organ system manages the flow of air into and out of your body. It oversees a number of vital body functions, including

✔ **Ventilating:** *Ventilation* — the act of breathing — isn't the same as *respiration* — the exchange of gases. You don't have to think about performing either task, but ventilation involves the physical movement of your diaphragm muscle, rib cage, and lungs to draw air in and push air out of the body. See the "Discovering the Ins and Outs of Breathing" section later in this chapter for details.

✔ **Exchanging gasses:** The job of the respiratory system is to supply oxygen and remove carbon dioxide from the blood as it circulates through the body. Chapter 4 explains how the blood gets into and out of the lungs in the process of *pulmonary circulation,* which is sometimes called *external respiration* to distinguish it from *cellular respiration.* Gas exchange happens in the lungs, where the respiratory tissues and the circulatory tissues meet. Refer to the later section "Respiratory membrane" to read more.

✔ **Regulating blood pH:** Maintaining blood pH within the homeostatic range requires coordination between the respiratory and urinary systems, with help from the endocrine system and, of course, the circulatory system itself.

✔ **Producing speech:** The ability of humans to consciously control breathing permits speech and singing.

Nosing around Your Respiratory Anatomy

The *respiratory tract* is the path of air from the nose to the lungs. It's divided into two sections: the *upper* respiratory tract (from the beginning of the airway at the nostrils to the pharynx) and the *lower* respiratory tract (from the top of the trachea to the diaphragm).

The respiratory tract is one of the places in the body where cells are replaced constantly throughout life.

We introduce you to each component of the human respiratory system in the sections that follow.

An entrance to the system: The nose

This is one time you can turn your nose up at your anatomy. Really. Point your nose up while looking in the mirror. (Yes, you have to put the book down.) See the two big openings?

Those are your *nostrils,* and they're two places where air enters and exits your respiratory system. Now, see all those tiny hairs in your nostrils? Those little hairs serve a purpose. They trap dirt, dust particles, and bacteria. Okay. You can put your head down now. The rest of your respiratory parts are way inside of your body, so you can't see them in the mirror.

Just beyond your nostrils, the *nasal septum* separates your *nasal cavities.* Inside the nasal cavities, the three tiny bones of the *nasal conchae* provide more surface area inside the nose because they're rolled up (like conch shells). The cells of the *respiratory mucosa* that lines the inside of the nasal cavity have tiny *cilia* that move the dirt-laden mucus toward the outside of the nostrils.

The *lacrimal glands* secrete tears that flow across the eye's surface and drain through the openings in the corner of the eye (*lacrimal puncta*), into the *nasolacrimal ducts* and the nasal cavities. That's why your nose runs when you cry.

Your *sinuses* are air spaces in your skull that lighten the weight of your head. They open into the nasal cavities so they can receive air as you breathe, and, like the nasal cavities, they're lined with mucous membranes.

Passing through the pharynx

Air passes through your *pharynx* on its way to your lungs. Along the way, it passes through and by some other important structures, such as your larynx and tonsils.

Your pharynx is divided into three regions based on what structures open into it:

- ✔ **Nasopharynx:** This is the top part of your throat where your nasal cavities drain. If you press your tongue to the roof of your mouth, you can feel your *hard palate.* This bony plate separates your mouth (*oral cavity*) from your nose (*nasal cavities*). If you move your tongue backward along the roof of your mouth, you reach a soft spot. This spot is the *soft palate.* Beyond the soft palate is your *nasopharynx,* which is where your nasal cavities drain into your throat. Your soft palate moves backward when you swallow so the nasopharynx is blocked.

Normally, the soft palate blocking the nasopharynx keeps food from going up into your nose. But when you're laughing and eating or drinking at the same time, your soft palate gets confused. When you go to swallow, it starts to move back, but when you laugh suddenly, it thrusts forward, allowing whatever's in your mouth to flow up into your nasal cavities and immediately fly out of your nostrils to the delight of everyone around you.

✔ **Oropharynx:** This is the middle part of your throat, but it's frequently referred to as the back of the throat. The oropharynx extends from the *uvula* to the level of the *hyoid bone.* It's the location of the *epiglottis,* a cartilage structure that guides materials passing though the mouth to the trachea or esophagus, as appropriate. This part of anatomy is the reason your food comes close to your windpipe but rarely goes in.

✔ **Laryngopharynx:** This is the lower part of your throat adjacent to your larynx. The *larynx* (or *voice box*) is triangular. At the apex of the triangle is *thyroid cartilage,* commonly known as your *Adam's apple.* If you could look down your throat onto the top of your larynx, you'd see your *glottis,* the opening through which air passes. When you swallow, a flap of tissue called your *epiglottis* covers your glottis and blocks food from getting into your larynx.

Inside your glottis are the *vocal cords* — gathered mucous membranes that cover ligaments. Your vocal cords vibrate when air passes over them, producing sound waves. Pushing more air over them increases the vibration's amplitude, making the sound louder. When you tighten your vocal cords, the glottis narrows, and your voice has a higher pitch.

Winding through the windpipe, or trachea

Your *trachea* (windpipe) is a tube that runs from your larynx to just above your lungs. Just behind your sternum, your trachea divides into two large branches called *primary bronchi* (singular, *bronchus*) that enter each lung.

The trachea and bronchi are made of smooth muscle and cartilage, allowing the airways to constrict and expand.

The lungs: The pair that just don't quit

Your lungs are large paired organs within your chest cavity on either side of your heart. Like the heart, they're protected by the rib cage. The lungs sit on top of the *diaphragm,* a powerful muscle that's fixed to the lower ribs, sternum, and lumbar vertebrae. The heart sits in a depression between the lungs, called the *cardiac notch.*

The right lung is somewhat larger than the left. Both lungs are separated into *lobes* (three on the right and two on the left). The lobes are further divided into segments and then into *lobules,* the smallest subdivision visible to the eye.

The following sections discuss two important lung-related structures.

Getting to know the pleural sac

Each lung is completely enclosed in the *pleural sac.* This sac is similar to the pericardial sac (which surrounds the heart) in that it's made up of two membranes, the *parietal* pleura, attached to the thoracic wall, and the *visceral* pleura, attached to the lung's surface, with the pleural cavity between them. The pleural cavity contains a lubricating fluid called the *intrapleural fluid.*

The intrapleural fluid completely surrounds the lungs. It keeps the pleural membranes moist and lubricated. Because this fluid has a pressure lower than atmospheric pressure (that is, little air is in the fluid), the lungs stay inflated.

Because of the adhesive force of the fluid interface between the parietal pleura and the visceral pleura, the lung is essentially attached to the chest wall. Thus, as muscles associated with the thoracic wall contract and relax and the chest rises and falls, the lungs expand and contract.

The visceral pleura surrounds the *mediastinum,* the region that separates the left and right lungs and houses the heart, thymus, and part of the esophagus.

Understanding the bronchial tree

After the primary bronchus enters the lung on each side, it splits into secondary and tertiary branches called *bronchi*. The tertiary bronchi divide into smaller branches called *brionchioles*. At the end of the smallest bronchioles are little structures that look like raspberries. These are the *alveolar sacs,* and each sac contains many *alveoli* (singular, *alveolus*). The alveoli's walls are composed of a simple squamous epithelium (designed to facilitate rapid diffusion) and elastic tissue that alternately stretches and constricts as you breathe.

Each of the approximately 300 million alveoli is wrapped with capillaries, whose walls, like the alveoli's walls, contains simple squamous epithelium, a tissue type adapted for the exchange of materials. The interface of the simple squamous epithelium of an alveolus and the simple squamous epithelium of a pulmonary capillary (along with its supporting connective tissue) is called the *respiratory membrane.* Gas exchange occurs in this membrane.

Exchanging gases at the respiratory membrane

The *respiratory membrane* refers to the area within the lung where the epithelial cells of the alveoli meet the capillaries and gas exchange takes place. Because of the folds and convolutions of the bronchioles and alveoli, the respiratory membrane has a large surface area. And because gas exchange for a large, active, warm-blooded animal requires a membrane with a large surface area, evolution has favored those with convoluted bronchioles and alveoli. Look to Figure 5-1 to get an understanding of the respiratory membrane's structure.

The respiratory membrane is the location where blood is reoxygenated in the process of pulmonary circulation, which we describe in detail in Chapter 4. The process of gas exchange at the respiratory membrane is almost exactly the same as the capillary exchange process, also covered in Chapter 4. However, at the respiratory membrane, oxygen flows through the alveolar wall and into the blood, and carbon dioxide flows out of the blood and through the alveolar wall into the air space. This process proceeds in the opposite direction of the flow in the capillary beds.

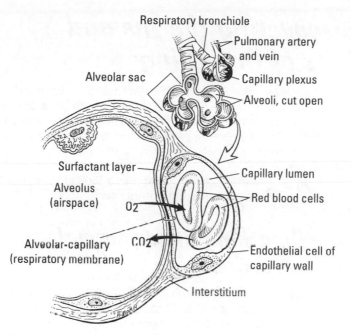

Respiratory bronchiole

Pulmonary artery and vein

Alveolar sac

Capillary plexus

Alveoli, cut open

Surfactant layer

Capillary lumen

Alveolus (airspace)

O_2

Red blood cells

Alveolar-capillary (respiratory membrane)

CO_2

Endothelial cell of capillary wall

Interstitium

Figure 5-1: Respiratory gases are exchanged by diffusion across alveolar and capillary walls.

The respiratory membrane is where carbon dioxide, the waste product of aerobic metabolism, is eliminated. It flows into the air in your lungs and you just breathe it out.

The comptroller of ventilation: The diaphragm

The *thoracic diaphragm* is a dome-shaped sheet of muscle separating the base of the lungs from the liver, and, on the left side, from the stomach and the spleen. The diaphragm pushes up beneath the lungs to control their contraction and expansion during ventilation. The motor fibers in the *phrenic nerves* signal to the diaphragm when to contract and relax. The diaphragm can also exert pressure on the abdominal cavity, helping with the expulsion of vomit, feces, or urine.

Discovering the Ins and Outs of Breathing

Breathing is essential to life, and thankfully, your body does it automatically. Air is alternately pulled into (inhaled) and pushed out of (exhaled) the lungs due to changes in the gas pressure in the alveoli. This change in pressure comes about because the alveoli are expanded when the chest cavity expands.

In the following sections, we take a look at how your body breathes under different conditions.

Breathing under normal conditions

When you're sleeping, sitting still, and doing normal activities, your breathing rate is 12 to 20 inhalation/exhalation cycles per minute. That's 17,000 breaths or more a day.

Normal breathing *(eupnea)* is involuntary, which is why you never really forget to breathe. Breathing continues during sleep. In many cases, breathing continues even during a coma. Impulses to the diaphragm come through a pair of spinal nerves, called the *phrenic nerves*. They initiate the regular alternating contraction and release of the diaphragm. The rhythm of the impulse is controlled by the autonomic system in the brain stem. (You can control your breath voluntarily, but doing so involves the cerebral cortex.)

Inspiration and expiration are the two processes that make up normal breathing. Here's the lowdown on each:

✔ **Inspiration:** *Inspiration* (breathing in) is the result of the diaphragm's contraction. The diaphragm moves downward into the abdomen, expanding the lungs as it does so. This, of course, decreases the air pressure in the lungs. (**Remember:** The diaphragm is attached to the base of the lungs at the bottom and the thoracic wall at the sides.) The skeletal muscles of the ribs (*intercostal* muscles) help to expand the lungs by pulling the ribs up and out. Air is pulled in at the top of the airway (nose and mouth) and all the way down to take up the expanded space in the alveoli.

✔ **Expiration:** *Expiration* (breathing out) is a passive process that occurs between impulses. Stretch receptors within the alveoli send nerve impulses to the respiratory center to release the contraction of the diaphragm. As the diaphragm relaxes, it moves back up out of the abdomen (because of abdominal muscle tone), the elastic tissue in the lungs snaps back (gets smaller), and the rib cage falls back (mostly because of gravity). This increases the air pressure in the lungs and pushes the air out (see Figure 5-2).

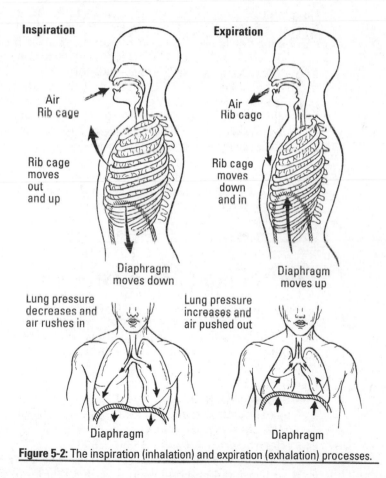

Figure 5-2: The inspiration (inhalation) and expiration (exhalation) processes.

Seeing how stress affects breathing

Breathing under stress is a bit different from breathing normally. Keep in mind that "stress" just means that an extra physiological demand is being placed on the body. Stress isn't necessarily negative — whether physical or emotional, stress can be painful or pleasurable, and it's often both.

No matter how much fun you are or aren't having, stress increases metabolism. More oxygen is consumed, and more carbon dioxide is produced. *Chemoreceptor cells* in the carotid arteries and aorta detect an elevated level of carbon dioxide or hydrogen ions and alert your respiratory center. Both inspiration and expiration become active processes. You breathe more deeply and frequently. The intercostal muscles forcefully contract and push more air out of your lungs (this can't occur during rest). These processes restore homeostasis and support the elevated metabolism.

The forcible exhalation involved in coughing or sneezing is aided by the sudden contraction of the abdominal muscles, raising the abdominal pressure. The rapid increase in pressure pushes the relaxed diaphragm up against the pleural cavity, forcing air out of the lungs.

Controlling your breathing

As far as has been determined, humans are the only animals who can bring their breathing under conscious control. Controlled breathing allows people to speak and sing as well as moderate other physiological systems. The following sections show you how.

Holding your breath

You can stop breathing (by holding your breath), at least for awhile, when unpleasant odors, noxious chemicals, or particulate matter is in the air around you, while you swim underwater, or just for the fun of it. The cerebral cortex sends signals to the rib muscles and the diaphragm that temporarily override the respiratory center signals.

Holding your breath long enough to cause damage to your own brain from a lack of oxygen isn't possible. Metabolism and gas exchange continue as usual while you hold your breath. Carbon dioxide concentration increases in the blood. At a certain point, long before brain damage is even a possibility, the chemoreceptors that work with the respiratory center are stimulated to the point where they override the cerebral cortex. At the extreme, you lose consciousness. (The evolutionarily older brainstem puts the whippersnapper cerebral cortex into time out.) You exhale and the system rapidly returns to normal.

Speaking and singing

Speech, another uniquely human activity, requires breath control. The exhalation passes breath over the vocal cords, causing sound waves to be emitted, and the lips and tongue shape the sound waves into speech. The rate of exhalation is lower while you're speaking and is controlled by the diaphragm, the intercostal muscles, and the abdominal muscles. Singing requires even more breath control than speaking.

Directing other systems

The relationship between the autonomic nervous system and the respiratory system appears to be two-way. For example, anxiety prompts hyperventilation, and hyperventilation produces symptoms of anxiety. Consciously controlling the rate and depth of breathing, mainly by achieving awareness and control of the diaphragm, has been demonstrated to decrease anxiety and sympathetic nervous system activation.

Controlled breathing is a feature of many religious, spiritual, and physical disciplines in all traditions. Clinical benefits have been demonstrated for meditation and controlled breathing in a wide variety of conditions of the neural, cardiovascular, and pulmonary systems.

Chapter 6

Getting on Track with the Digestive System

*J*ust how does that meal of steak, potatoes, and salad become the tissues of your body? The digestive organ system gets it halfway there. (The circulatory system, which we cover in Chapter 4, does most of the rest.)

Living systems constantly exchange energy. Physiological processes — anabolic, catabolic, and homeostatic — require energy. Ultimately, that energy comes from the light energy that plants use to transform carbon in the atmosphere (as CO_2) into biological matter (as carbohydrate) in the process of *photosynthesis*. Humans get their energy by consuming this biological matter, either directly or by consuming other organisms that do. The digestive system takes apart this biological matter step by step and transforms it into a form that human cells can use. In this chapter, we explain the ins and outs of the process and the organs responsible for the chore.

Your Digestive System in a Nutshell

Digestion itself is a middle step. Other important functions of this organ system come before and after:

✔ **Ingesting:** Although all animals *ingest* — take something into the body through the mouth — only humans, and possibly some of the great apes, appear to enjoy food as they ingest it.

The perception of subtle flavors is more closely connected to olfaction than digestion. The perception of the five basic flavors is also considered *neurosensory*. Perception in the mouth is more about texture and is closely related to food's protein and fat content. This concept is captured by the food industry term *mouth feel*. These sensory perceptions guide you in the selection of foods.

Sometimes, though, ingestion isn't a feast for the senses — nothing delicious is available. The body still needs calories, though, so whatever's available is chewed and swallowed just the same.

✔ **Digesting:** Eating is fun, and ingestion is bearable, but neither provides biological molecules that your cells can use. That task is accomplished by the interaction of physical and chemical forces. The digestive tract is a muscular tube lined with chemical factories that operate under the direction of their own dedicated neural structures and under hormonal control.

The digestive system processes everything down the same track, extracting fuel, biological molecules and monomers, and micronutrients from whatever you eat. (See the section "Importing and Exporting: The intestines," later in this chapter.)

✔ **Exporting nutrients to the body:** The end products of digestion are biological molecules, such as glucose, that are absorbed across the digestive membrane into the blood and then distributed in the body.

✔ **Eliminating:** The elimination of digestive waste is part of digestion. Other organ systems have evolved to make use of the digestive system's structures to eliminate metabolic wastes of other kinds.

Moving through the Structures of the Digestive Tract

The *digestive tract*, also called the *alimentary canal* (*alimentary* means food), or the *gastrointestinal (GI) tract*, is a tube through which ingested substances are pushed along for physical and chemical processing. The tube walls are made up of an outer fibrous layer, a muscular layer, a supportive connective tissue layer, and an inner layer (containing an epithelial lining), called the *digestive mucosa.* All the layers vary in thickness from one place to another along the digestive tract. The space inside the tube is the *lumen,* and its size varies, too.

The digestive system's gross anatomy (no pun here) is comparable to that of an industrial smelter. Some structures bring in raw materials; other structures extract, process, and ship out specific substances; and still other structures export the unused part of the raw materials back into the environment. The body uses both mechanical and chemical mechanisms to break down the raw materials and export products to the larger system (the economy in the case of the smelter; the organism in the case of the intestine). These efficient systems are organized linearly — things keep moving along in one direction at a steady pace.

In the following sections, we describe in detail each structure of the digestive tract and what it does to keep things moving through the digestive process.

Allowing entry: The mouth

Your mouth is the starting point of your digestive system, the gateway to your other digestive organs. Besides making eating a fun experience, your mouth (or *oral cavity,* for the technical term) serves some important digestive functions, as described in the next sections.

Teeth and gums for tearing and grinding

Humans have 32 teeth — 16 on the top and 16 on the bottom. Your teeth tear and grind food into pieces that are small enough to swallow, and they come in four basic types: incisors for biting, canines for tearing, and premolars and molars for grinding.

The *gingiva* (gums) hold teeth in position, and a binding material called *cementum* embeds your teeth's roots in your jawbone. Blood vessels that run through the jawbone and up into the pulp of the tooth supply the teeth with blood. *Dentin,* a bonelike material, covers the pulp, and an extremely hard protective enamel covers the dentin.

A tongue to help with chewing

Your tongue is mainly skeletal muscle tissue. The muscle is covered on the upper surface by a mucous membrane, in which are embedded taste buds. The tongue muscles move the food around in your mouth to assist chewing. The mucus moistens and lubricates the *bolus,* the technical term for a mouthful of food in the process of being chewed.

Muscles attach your tongue to your skull bones, and a mucous membrane on the tongue's underside attaches your tongue to the oral cavity floor. That stringy piece of membrane that you see when you touch your tongue's tip to the roof of your mouth is the *lingual frenulum.*

The buccal membrane to kick-start digestion

The *buccal membrane* is that portion of the digestive mucosa that lines the inside of the mouth. Several *salivary glands* have ducts that course through the buccal membrane and secrete mucus and *salivary amylase,* a digestive enzyme, into the oral cavity. These glands often go into action before you take the first bite of your meal. A delicious aroma or even just the anticipation of eating something you enjoy can get those juices flowing.

Sending food to the stomach: The pharynx and esophagus

The *pharynx,* better known as your throat, leads to the *esophagus,* the tube that extends from the mouth to the stomach. When you swallow, the bolus bounces off a piece of cartilage called the *epiglottis* and is diverted from the *trachea* (which we tell you about in Chapter 5) and into the esophagus (see Figure 6-1).

The esophagus has two sphincters — one at the top and one at the bottom — that control the movement of the bolus into and out of the esophagus. The *pharyngoesophageal sphincter,* composed of skeletal muscle, takes part in the muscular actions involved in swallowing. Peristalsis propels the bolus along the esophagus. The lower esophageal sphincter surrounds the esophagus just as it enters the stomach.

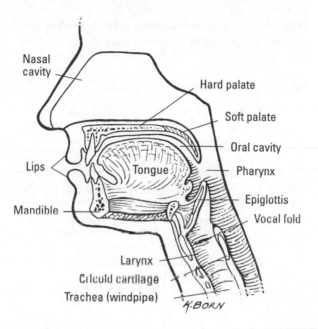

Figure 6-1: Structures of the mouth and pharynx.

Lining it up: The walls

The upper third of the esophagus is made of skeletal muscle. Beginning in the middle third of the esophagus and extending to the *anal sphincter,* layers of smooth muscle line the digestive tract. This smooth muscle contracts in pulsating waves, pushing the lumen's contents along in a single direction. This constant wave like contraction is called *peristalsis.*

A mucous membrane lines the digestive system, running continuously from the mouth all the way through to the rectum. This membrane protects your digestive organs from the strong acids and powerful enzymes secreted in the digestive system. The membrane's innermost cells (next to the lumen) are among those cells that are continuously replaced.

The digestive mucosa's secretions keep everything in the digestive tract moist, soft, and slippery, protecting the membrane and its underlying structures from abrasion and corrosion. The digestive mucosa contains tissues and cells that secrete other substances as well, including gastric acid, hormones, neurotransmitters, and enzymes. The digestive mucosa also contains an extensive network of lymphatic tissue.

Breaking it all down: The stomach

After passing through the bottom sphincter of the esophagus, the bolus drops into the stomach, the widest and most flexible part of the alimentary canal. Food remains in the stomach about two to six hours, during which it's churned in an acidic substance that the stomach secretes called *gastric juice,* ground up by thousands of strong muscle contractions, and offered in tiny pieces to protein-digesting enzymes.

The outside of the stomach is a tough connective tissue layer called the *serosa.* Beneath the serosa is the *muscular coat,* which has three layers of smooth muscle fibers — oblique, circular, and longitudinal — that contract in different directions. Stretch receptors in this layer send nerve impulses to the brain when the stomach is full. These two layers support the structure of the stomach as a hollow organ.

Beneath these connective tissue layers are two mucosal layers, the *submucosal coat* and the *mucous coat,* also called the *stomach lining.* Gastric glands in the mucosa secrete the components of gastric juice. The mucosal coat is corrugated, increasing the surface area inside the hollow. The folds are called *rugae.* As the stomach fills, the rugae smooth out, allowing the stomach to expand.

The stomach's muscular action is part of physical digestion, like chewing, swallowing, and peristalsis. But the stomach's contribution to chemical digestion is what really helps break down the food you eat.

As the stomach churns the bolus in the gastric acid, the material turns into an oatmeal-like paste called *chyme.* The chyme squirts into the small intestine through the *pyloric sphincter,* between the lower part of the stomach, called the *pylorus,* and the top of the small intestine, called the *duodenum.*

Importing and exporting: The intestines

The *intestine* is a long muscular tube (up to about 20 feet, or 6 meters) that extends from the pyloric sphincter to the anal sphincter. How does 20 feet of tubing fit into a relatively small space that's also crowded with other organs? It becomes narrow and convoluted. The intestines are classified as small and large based on their width, not their length (like hoses). The lumen of the small intestine is about 1 inch (2.5 centimeters) in diameter; the large intestine is about 2.5 inches (6.4 centimeters).

Overall, the intestine specializes in the import and export of biological substances of many kinds. As is usual for organs with import-export functions, the intestine has structures that maximize the surface area available for the exchange.

The intestine's muscular outer walls lie coiled closely together within the abdominal cavity, held in place by the fibrous sheets of the *peritoneum*. With two layers of smooth muscle tissue, longitudinal and circular, the intestine specializes in strong, sustained peristalsis.

The intestinal mucosa is continuous with the rest of the digestive mucosa. It's studded with specialized "work areas" that produce hormones, neurotransmitters, enzymes, and other substances integral to the digestive process.

The capillary beds that line the intestine define the interface of the digestive and circulatory systems. These capillaries are arrayed more or less continuously along the intestine's lumen.

The lumen is lined by *villi* (singular, *villus*), a structure that's specialized for import and export processes and that's characteristic of tissues in body locations where substances are exchanged. *Villi* are fingerlike projections of the mucosa that multiply the surface area available for exchange, much like wharves and piers extending into a harbor increase the area for harbor activities.

Villi line the entire length of the small intestine, projecting out into the lumen. Each villus has its own assigned capillary for absorbing materials from the intestine into the blood (flip to Chapter 4 for more on the circulatory system). *Microvilli* are even smaller projections on the epithelial cells of the mucosa.

Some of these processes require *active transport* — the expenditure of some energy in the form of ATP (see Chapter 2).

The following sections focus in on the specific jobs of both the small and large intestines.

Investigating the small intestine

The small intestine does a lot of the physical work of the digestive system, beginning with peristalsis. It's also majorly involved in digestive chemistry.

The small intestine is an endocrine gland as well as a digestive organ, producing and secreting hormones that control digestion. Cells in the small intestine's walls secrete the hormones *secretin* and *cholecystokinin* (CCK), which stimulate the release of digestive fluids, such as bile, from the gallbladder and pancreatic juice from the pancreas.

The small intestine's walls are lined with secretory tissue that functions in chemical digestion. Cells in the duodenum's walls secrete digestive enzymes. *Brunner's glands* in the small intestine's lining secrete mucus and bicarbonate directly into the lumen to help neutralize the gastric juice in the chyme. (Most enzymes require a near-neutral pH.)

The small intestine is divided into three structures along its 10-to-20-foot (3-to-6-meter) length: the *duodenum* (about 1 foot long, or 0.3 meters), the *jejunum* (about 3 to 6 feet, or 1 to 2 meters), and the *ileum* (about 6 to 12 feet, or 2 to 4 meters). The small intestine is approximately 1 to 2 inches (2.5 to 5 centimeters) in diameter.

Understanding the work of the large intestine

Chyme oozes from the small intestine to the large intestine (also called the *colon*), passing out of the ileum through the *ileocecal valve* into the *cecum,* the first portion of the large intestine. The material is now called *feces.*

The large intestine is about 6 feet long (almost 2 meters) and is positioned anatomically like a "frame" around the small intestine. Beyond the cecum, the large intestine moves upward as the *ascending colon,* across as the *transverse colon,* and downward as the *descending colon* and finally into the *sigmoid colon.*

In the large intestine, water is reabsorbed from the feces by diffusion across the intestinal wall into the capillaries. The removal of water compacts the indigestible material in the colon, forming the characteristic texture of the feces.

In addition to undigested food, the feces contain other bodily wastes to be excreted. The brown color of feces comes from the combination of greenish-yellow bile pigments, broken down hemoglobin, and bacteria.

Your intestines are home to unimaginably large numbers of bacteria, including hundreds of species. Trillions of tiny (pro- karyotic) cells ingest some of the undigested material in your feces, producing molecules that have a well-known odor. (It's nothing to be embarrassed about and nothing to be proud of, either.) Some of these bacteria produce beneficial substances, such as vitamin K, which is necessary for blood clotting. These substances are absorbed through the intestinal wall and transported into the blood via the capillaries.

Passing through the colon and rectum

As the colon completes its work, peristalsis moves feces into the *rectum*, which is located at the bottom of the colon. Stretch receptors in the rectum signal to the brain the need to defecate (release feces) when the rectum contains about 5 to 8 ounces (142 to 227 grams). Pushed by peristalsis, the feces pass through the *anal canal* and exit the body through the anal sphincter.

Doing the Chemical Breakdown

The liver and pancreas are often referred to as the *accessory organs of digestion*. They're not part of the digestive tract; they never come into contact with ingested material, and they take no part in the mechanical aspects of digestion. But they do produce and make available to the digestive tract's organs some of the chemical and biological substances that assist in digestion's chemical aspects.

We explore these organs and their function in the digestive process in the following sections.

The liver

The *liver* is one of the most important organs, not just in digestion but in many other functions. The liver's digestive function is the production and transport of *bile,* one of the digestive chemicals.

Many of the terms related to the liver's structures and functions contain the prefix *hepato-,* meaning "liver."

Liver anatomy

Your liver is both the largest internal organ and the largest gland in the human body. A healthy adult human liver weighs about 3 to 3.5 pounds (1.4 to 1.6 kilograms). It's located under your diaphragm and above your stomach on the right side of your abdomen (see Figure 6-2). The liver is soft, pinkish-brown, and triangular, with four lobes of unequal size and shape: the *right lobe, left lobe, quadrate lobe,* and *caudate lobe.* The liver is covered by a connective tissue capsule that branches and extends throughout its insides, providing a scaffolding of support for the afferent blood vessels, lymphatic vessels, and bile ducts that traverse it.

The liver receives oxygenated blood through the *hepatic artery,* which comes from the *aorta.* It receives nutrient-rich blood through the *portal vein,* which carries blood from the capillaries of the small intestine and the descending colon (see Chapter 4 for more on the circulatory system). Three hepatic veins drain deoxygenated blood from the liver, exiting the liver at the top of the right lobe and draining into the *inferior vena cava.*

Each of the four lobes is made up of tiny lobules, about 100,000 of them in all. The *hepatic lobule* is the liver's functional unit. Each lobule is made up of millions of hepatic cells and bile canals and is supported and separated by branches of the capsule. At the lobule's vertices are regularly distributed *portal triads* that contain a bile duct, a terminal branch of the hepatic artery, and a terminal branch of the portal vein. The *hepatocytes* are in a roughly hexagonal arrangement, with a vein in the center that carries the lobule's products out into the blood. On the surface of the lobules are ducts, veins, and arteries that carry fluids to and from them.

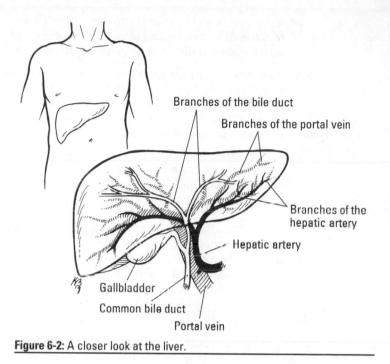

Branches of the bile duct

Branches of the portal vein

Branches of the hepatic artery

Hepatic artery

Gallbladder

Common bile duct

Portal vein

Figure 6-2: A closer look at the liver.

Bile production and transport

The liver produces bile, a major factor in the digestion of fats and lipids of all kinds. The bile that some of the lobules produce is collected in bile *canaliculi*, which merge to form *bile ducts*. The *intrahepatic* (within the liver) bile ducts eventually drain directly into the duodenum through the *common hepatic duct*.

Bile can also be transported for storage into the gallbladder via the *extrahepatic* bile ducts. Your *gallbladder* is a pear-shaped sac tucked into the curve of your liver whose only function is to store bile and deliver it on demand to the duodenum. The bile flows through the common bile duct into the duodenum, near the entry point of the *pancreatic duct*.

Other functions of the liver

The liver functions in many other ways, affecting other organ systems. Here's a brief overview of its many functions:

✔ It processes and eliminates toxins. Toxic byproducts of some drugs, including alcohol, and other substances arrive from the digestive organs through the portal vein.

✔ It processes and eliminates metabolic waste. The liver removes dying red blood cells from the blood and converts the hemoglobin to *bilirubin* and other byproducts. These are delivered to the intestine and excreted with the feces. (The iron is recycled.)

✔ It stores glucose in the form of *glycogen* and reconverts it when blood glucose levels get low. This function is mediated by insulin and glucagon.

✔ It stores vitamins and minerals.

✔ It produces many kinds of protein, including protein hormones, the plasma proteins, and the proteins of the clotting cascade and the complement system, as well as the production of alpha and beta globulin.

The pancreas

The *pancreas* sits in the abdominal cavity next to the duodenum and behind the stomach. It produces *pancreatic juice,* which is full of pancreatic enzymes that are important in digestion. Refer to Table 6-1 for information about pancreatic enzymes. Nearly every cell of the pancreas secretes pancreatic juice and passes it through the *pancreatic duct* into the duodenum.

Table 6-1	Pancreatic Enzymes	
Enzyme	*Targeted Nutrient*	*Result of Breakdown*
Trypsin	Proteins	Peptides (chains of amino acids)
Peptidase	Peptides	Individual amino acids
Lipase	Fats	Fatty acids and glycerol
Nuclease	Nucleic acids (DNA, RNA)	Nucleotides
Amylase	Carbohydrates	Glucose and fructose

The pancreas also produces the hormones *insulin* and *glucagon.* These hormones work to control the amount of glucose in the blood.

Insulin is released when the blood's glucose level rises. It acts by stimulating glucose uptake in cells. With plenty of glucose available, the cell's metabolic rate increases, and it produces more of its specialized anabolic product. Glucose is burned to fuel physiologically productive reactions. Insulin also stimulates glucose uptake activity in the energy storage cells in the liver, muscle cells, and fatty tissue.

A lower blood glucose level stimulates the pancreas to secrete insulin's partner glucagon, which pulls glucose from cells where it's stored and releases it into the blood. Glucagon keeps the metabolic fires burning at a steady level.

Digestive fluids, enzymes, and hormones

Each part of the digestive system has its characteristic fluid, each a complex mixture of water, electrolytes, and biological substances with a specific role in digestion.

- **Mucus:** Every inch of the digestive tract has mucus glands whose secretions keep everything in the digestive tract moist, soft, and slippery, protecting the digestive membrane and its underlying structures from abrasion and corrosion.

- **Saliva:** Saliva (or spit) is a clear, watery solution that the salivary glands in your mouth produce constantly. You produce about 2 to 4 pints (1 to 2 liters) of spit every day. Saliva moistens food and makes it easier to swallow. It's also a component of the sense of taste — a food substance must be dissolved in the watery solution for its chemical signals to act on your taste buds.

    Enzymes in saliva start starch digestion even before you swallow food. The combination of chewing food and coating it with saliva makes the tongue's job a bit easier — it can push wet, chewed food toward the throat more easily.

Saliva cleans the inside of your mouth and your teeth. The enzymes in saliva also help to fight off infections in the mouth.

✔ **Enzymes:** Thousands of enzymes are involved in digestion. Enzymes are specialized in their function — a given
enzyme typically catalyzes one or only a few specific
reactions. Digestive enzymes specialize in reactions that
break specific molecules apart into component chemical
entities. They can be broadly classified as *proteinases* and
peptidases, lipidases, and various kinds of *carbohydrate-
active* enzymes. Enzymes are part of the digestive fluids'
gastric juice and pancreatic juice.

The suffix *-ase* indicates an enzyme that breaks a molecule apart.

✔ **Gastric juice:** Gastric juice is secreted from millions of
tiny gastric glands in the gastric mucosa and enters the
hollow of the stomach through *gastric pits* on the mucosa's
inner surface. Gastric juice contains *hydrochloric acid*
(HCl), which is extremely acidic and kills bacteria that
may have entered the body with food. It also contains the
powerful proteinase *pepsin,* which can work only in this
highly acidic environment.

✔ **Pancreatic juice:** Pancreatic juice contains many types of
digestive enzymes. Refer to Table 6-1 for details.

✔ **Bile:** Bile, also called *gall,* is a very alkaline, bitter-tasting,
dark-green to yellowish-brown fluid produced by the
liver. Bile may remain in the liver or be transported to
the gallbladder for storage before being expelled into
the duodenum.

The physiological function of bile is to emulsify fats — that
is, to create an environment in which lipid-based substances can be mixed in a watery matrix for transportation and to make them available for chemical reactions to
break them down. Bile's high alkalinity helps neutralize
the strongly acidic chyme that comes into the duodenum
from the stomach. Another purpose of bile is to help
absorb the fat-soluble vitamins K, D, and A into the blood.

Chapter 7

Passing through the Urinary System

In This Chapter

▶ Understanding what the urinary system does

▶ Breaking down the urinary system's parts

▶ Ruminating on the role of urine

▶ Seeing how your body maintains homeostasis

Generally speaking, everything that enters your body through your digestive system must be excreted back into the environment in some form eventually. Most of the waste products of cellular metabolism and many other substances exit your body via your urinary system. Urine is the body's primary waste product, and urination (the release of urine to the environment) is the final step of metabolism.

In this chapter, we take you on a tour of the urinary system, reveal the makeup of urine, and explain how the kidneys help your body maintain homeostasis.

Running Down the Urinary System's Responsibilities

The functions of the human urinary system, as defined in the following list, are similar to those of typical reptiles, birds, and mammals, with some differences in the details.

✔ **Doing the dirty work:** Cellular metabolic wastes are toxic and would cause harm to the cell if they were allowed to accumulate. Cells, therefore, continuously export their metabolic wastes into the extracellular fluid. As extracellular fluid is absorbed into the venous blood during capillary exchange, the waste substances enter the circulatory system. Carbon dioxide is excreted in the lungs in the pulmonary circulation cycle. Other byproducts of cellular metabolism travel in the arterial (oxygenated) blood to the renal artery and into the kidney. The function of the urinary system is to remove these toxic byproducts from the blood and then eliminate them from the body.

The term *excretion* can mean the movement of material from the inside to the outside of a cell, as well as the release of material from the inside to the outside of the body.

✔ **Making and expelling urine:** *Urine* is a watery solution produced by your kidneys. It's the matrix through which the water-soluble waste products of metabolism, mainly nitrogenous metabolic byproducts, are removed from the blood and eliminated from the body. Urine also helps maintain the chemical equilibrium of the blood because substances harmful to the chemical equilibrium of the blood can be dumped there.

✔ **Balancing water content:** Around half of your body weight is water, contained in intracellular and extracellular fluid, the plasma of your blood, your lymph fluid, and the fluids in your digestive tract and mucous membranes. Your kidneys precisely regulate the release and retention of water to maintain blood volume, composition, and chemical variables within homeostatic ranges.

✔ **Performing endocrine functions:** The kidney is one of the most important endocrine organs. The adrenal endocrine glands are located on top of the kidneys but outside the kidney capsule, so they're not part of the kidneys. Many of the hormones produced and secreted by these glands act on the kidneys.

  • **Regulating RBC production:** The hormone *erythropoietin,* which regulates RBC (red blood cell) production *(erythropoiesis)* in the bone marrow, is produced in the *peritubular capillary endothelial cells* in the kidney and liver. Erythropoietin also has other physiological functions related to wound healing and recovery.

- **Regulating bone growth:** *Calcitriol,* the physiologically active form of vitamin D, is synthesized in the kidneys from a precursor molecule synthesized in the liver. Calcitriol regulates, among other things, the concentration of calcium and phosphate in the blood, which promotes the healthy mineralization, growth, and remodeling of bone.

Surveying the Structures of the Urinary System

The human urinary system is quite compact. Unlike some other organ systems, you can identify the point where it begins and another point, not too far away, where it ends.

Like the alimentary canal, the *urinary system* is essentially a system of tubes through which a substance passes, undergoing a series of physiological processes as it does so. The familiar tissue layers — an outer fibrous covering, a muscular layer, and a mucous layer lining the interior surface — are seen throughout the urinary system, beginning at the ureter. The mucus protects the tissues from the caustic urine.

The following sections get you acquainted with the various parts of the urinary system.

Creating urine: The kidneys

The urinary system begins with the *kidneys,* fist-sized paired organs that are reddish-brown in color and located just below the ribs in your lower back. A single kidney is shaped like an elongated oval; actually, it's shaped just like a kidney bean. (Coincidence?) The inner curve of the kidney has a large concavity (depression) called the *hilum* where a number of vessels enter or exit, including the ureter, renal artery, renal vein, lymphatic vessels, and nerves. A connective tissue membrane called the *peritoneum,* as well as adipose (fat) tissue, attach your kidneys to your posterior abdominal wall. (The term *renal* comes from the Latin *ren,* meaning "kidney.")

Beneath the peritoneum, a lining of collagen called the *capsule* encloses the kidney. Fibers of this layer extend outward to attach the organ to surrounding structures.

Renal blood supply

The *renal artery,* a large branch of the abdominal aorta, brings blood into the kidney for filtering. The renal vein drains filtered blood out of the kidney. The kidneys receive about 20 percent of all blood pumped by the heart each minute.

Kidney tissues

Under the capsule, the kidney's various tissues are arranged in more or less concentric layers. The outermost layer, just beneath the capsule, is the *cortex.* Beneath the cortex is the *medulla,* a series of fan-shaped structures comprising a membrane that's convoluted (folded) into conical structures, called *renal pyramids,* that secrete urine at their tips into sac-like structures. The innermost layer is the *renal pelvis,* which channels the urine from these sacs into the *ureter.*

Nephron

Microscopic in size (about a million of them exist in each kidney), the *nephron* is the kidney's filtering unit. Each nephron has two parts: the *renal corpuscle* and the *renal tubule.* The renal corpuscle also has two parts: the *glomulerus* (plural, *glomeruli*), a special kind of capillary bed derived from arterioles branching from the renal artery, and the *glomerular capsule* or *Bowman's capsule,* a double-walled epithelial cup that partially encloses the glomerulus.

Leading away from the capsule, the nephron loops up, forming the *proximal convoluted tubule,* or PCT. The tube then straightens, pushing down into the medulla and looping up again (the *loop of Henle*). At the top, it loops again into the *distal convoluted tubule* (DCT). This tubule connects with a collecting duct that carries the urine through the renal pyramids into a series of sac-like structures in the renal pelvis.

The nephrons are surrounded by the *peritubular capillaries,* which perform an important role in direct secretion, selective reabsorption, and the regulation of water.

Make sure you keep the *kidney capsule* and the *glomerular capsules* straight. The kidney has one kidney capsule on the outside and a million microscopic glomerular capsules inside.

Holding and releasing: The urinary tract

All complex animals have evolved ways of removing metabolic waste and regulating water balance, but only mammals have evolved an organ, the bladder, for sequestering urine so it may be excreted voluntarily. Whatever the evolutionary imperative that caused the development of this part of the mammalian urinary system, some groups have developed chemical signaling mechanisms that utilize it. For humans, the ability to control the time and place of urination may be crucial for their ability to live in dense groups.

The *urinary tract* is the name of the part of the urinary system from the top of the ureter to the external urethral opening, the route of urine out of the body. It consists of the ureters, bladder, and urethra.

Ureters

The *ureters* are tubes that transport urine from a kidney to the bladder. The ureter emerges from the renal pelvis.

The walls of the ureter are similar in structure to those of the intestines: The muscular layer contracts in waves of peristalsis to move urine from the kidney to the bladder.

Bladder

The *bladder* is a hollow, funnel-shaped sac into which urine flows from the kidneys through the ureters. The bladder has a capacity of about 20 ounces (about three-fifths of a liter). It lies in the pelvic cavity, just behind the pubic bones and centered in front of the rectum. In females, it's in front of the uterus and vagina.

Like other organs in the urinary and digestive systems, the bladder is made up of an outer protective membrane, several layers of muscles arranged in opposing directions, and an inner mucosal layer. The muscle layers contract to expel urine into the urethra. The mucosa is made up of a special kind of epithelial tissue called *transitional epithelium* in which the cells can change shape from columnar to squamous to accommodate larger volumes of urine (see Figure 7-1). Pressure (stretch) receptors in the muscle layer send impulses to the brain when the bladder is becoming full.

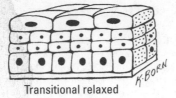

Transitional relaxed

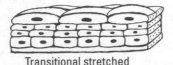

Transitional stretched

Figure 7-1: Transitional epithelium lines the bladder. _____

Urethra

The *urethra* is a tube that carries urine from the bladder to an opening (orifice) of the body for elimination. The *mucosa* (epithelium) of the urethra is composed of transitional cells as it exits the bladder. Farther along are stratified columnar cells, followed by stratified squamous cells near the external urethral orifice. Mucus from small glands in the mucosa help protect the epithelium from the corrosive urine.

In both males and females, a sphincter at the proximal end of the urethra (between the bladder and the urethra) retains urine in the bladder. This sphincter, called the *internal urethral sphincter,* is made of smooth muscle and is under the control of the autonomic nervous system. It opens to release urine into the urethra.

Where the urethra traverses the *urogenital diaphragm* (the floor of the pelvis), there's a sphincter made of striated fibers (skeletal muscle) called the *external urethral sphincter,* which is under voluntary control.

The male and female urethrae are adapted to interact with the respective reproductive systems (which we cover in Chapter 8) and, therefore, differ from each other in some aspects of anatomy and physiology.

✔ **Female urethra:** In females, the urethra is about 1.5 inches (3.8 centimeters) long, from its point of emergence from the bladder to the urethral orifice. It runs along the anterior wall of the vagina and opens between the clitoris and the vaginal orifice. The external sphincter is located just inside the exit point.

✔ **Male urethra:** In males, the urethra is about 8 inches (20 centimeters) long, from its point of emergence from the bladder to its opening at the tip of the penis, called the *urethral meatus*. As it passes through the prostate gland and the penis, the male urethra is divided into three named sections, based on anatomical structures:

- The *prostatic urethra* contains the internal sphincter and passes through the prostate. Openings in this region allow for the passage of sperm and prostatic fluid into the urethra during orgasm.

- The *membranous urethra* contains the external sphincter. It's only about 1 inch (2.5 centimeters) in length.

- The *cavernous urethra,* or *spongy urethra,* runs the length of the penis on its ventral surface, ending at the urethral meatus.

The Yellow River

Urine is a bodily fluid with specific functions, just like blood and lymph. But unlike those, you see urine in the normal course of everyday events. Here's everything you always wanted to know about how it gets to be its own sweet self.

Looking at the composition of urine

Urine is about 95 percent water, in which is dissolved urea, other nitrogenous compounds, and varying concentrations of electrolytes, plus assorted inorganic and organic compounds. Its odor comes from ammonia and other substances derived from ammonia, such as urea. See Table 7-1 for more about the nitrogenous components of urine.

Table 7-1	Nitrogenous Components of Urine and Their Sources
Nitrogenous Component	**Source**
Urea	A byproduct of the breakdown of amino acids
Creatinine	A byproduct of the metabolism of the amino acid *creatine,* present in large quantities in muscle cells
Ammonia	A byproduct of the breakdown of proteins by bacteria
Uric acid	A byproduct of the breakdown of *nucleotides*

Urine is yellow because it contains *urobilinogen,* a compound formed from the breakdown of red blood cells. The normal color range of urine is some shade of yellow, from nearly clear to dark amber, depending mostly on one's level of hydration. When you're abundantly hydrated, lots of water goes into the urine, making it more diluted and, therefore, paler. When you're less than optimally hydrated, the kidneys put less water into the urine. As a result, the urine becomes more concentrated and appears darker.

Ingested food, beverages, and pharmaceutical products influence the composition of urine. Urine contains *hippuric acid,* produced by the digestion of fruits and vegetables, and *ketone bodies,* produced by the digestion of fats. Some foods, beverages, and drugs impart color and odor to urine. Some physiological conditions and disorders affect the composition of urine, and urine has long been analyzed for clinical signs.

To maintain the blood pH within the homeostatic range (7.3 to 7.4), the kidney can produce urine with a pH as low as 4.5 or as high as 8.5.

Filtering the blood

The glomerulus and the glomerular capsule make up the area of interface between the circulatory system and the kidney. That's where your body filters blood.

The blood pressure in these capillaries is higher than in other capillaries, and it pushes the blood up against the glomerular wall with some force. Because it's a process that relies on mechanical force (fluid pressure), glomerular filtration separates particles based on one criterion: molecule size.

The thin, permeable glomerular wall acts as a filtration membrane. Water passes through into the capsule, bringing along small-molecule solutes, including wastes and toxins like urea and creatinine and useful small-molecule substances such as glucose, amino acids, and electrolyte ions. Large solutes, such as proteins and nutrients, remain in the plasma inside the glomerular vessel and continue on in the circulating blood. The watery solution (filtrate) passes into the top of the renal tubule at the capsule.

Reabsorbing selectively

An important aspect of urine production is the restoration of glucose, amino acids, and electrolyte ions, not to mention water, from the filtrate to the blood. As the filtrate passes along the nephron, it's acted upon by different types of specialized tissue. Processes in the following specialized tissues are responsible for the composition of urine:

- **Microvilli:** *Microvilli* line the nephrons, increasing the surface area within the tubule where substances can enter and leave the filtrate.

- **PCT:** Na (sodium ion) undergoes active transport from the filtrate to the blood at the PCT. Where Na+ goes, Cl– just naturally follows. This situation creates an osmotic pressure gradient that pulls water out of the filtrate and into the blood. Approximately 65 percent of the water and salts are returned to the blood at the PCT.

  Some substances, including K+ and some hormones, are secreted from the adjacent *peritubular capillaries* into the PCT. This process is termed *direct secretion*.

- **Loop of Henle:** At the loop of Henle, electrolytes and urea move out of the nephron into the medulla. The filtrate remaining in the nephron, now *urine,* drains through the DCT into the collecting duct and then into the renal pelvis.

- **Medulla:** The solutes that enter the medulla from the loop of Henle draw water into the medulla. Capillaries in the medulla restore some of the water to the blood.

✔ **DCT:** Active transport passes amino acids, glucose, and electrolytes (those useful substances that happen to be small enough to pass through the filtration membrane) back into the blood at the DCT. Water reabsorption at the DCT occurs under the control of ADH.

✔ **Collecting duct:** Reabsorption of water occurs in the collecting duct. As salts are reabsorbed, water follows. The amount of water reabsorbed from the filtrate back into the blood depends on the hydration situation in the body. However, even in cases of extreme dehydration, the kidneys produce around 16 ounces (about half a liter) of urine per day just to excrete toxic waste substances.

Numerous other substances are returned to the blood at specific points, conserving them and maintaining the blood's chemical environment. More than 99 percent of the filtrate produced each day can be reabsorbed. The processes are called *selective reabsorption* because the details are different for (chemically) different types of substances.

Expelling urine

Urine drips down the nephron's collecting ducts to the renal pelvis. From there, it moves along the ureter and into the bladder. As the urine accumulates, the pressure receptors in the lining send signals to the brain. The first message is sent when the bladder is about half full (around 6 to 8 ounces, or 177 to 237 milliliters). At a volume of 12 ounces (354 milliliters), the messages become stronger, and it becomes difficult to control the external urethral sphincter.

When the time is right to empty the bladder, the brain sends an impulse through the autonomic nervous system to open the internal urethral sphincter and contract the bladder muscles. Urine flows out of the bladder, through the urethra, and out of the body.

Maintaining Homeostasis

The chemistry of life, stunningly complex and precise, requires a tightly controlled environment to proceed optimally. The kidneys, under hormonal control, are key organs for maintaining the chemical homeostasis of blood and other body fluids. The endocrine system has a huge range of subtle and interacting mechanisms for controlling kidney function. (See Chapter 9 for the scoop on the endocrine system.)

Connecting fluid balance and blood pressure

Aspects of fluid balance that involve the blood include blood volume and the amount and nature of the electrolytes in the plasma. These factors are linked, as we explain in the following sections.

Blood volume (water content)

The concentration of *electrolytes* (ions), such as Na+, Cl–, and K+, helps determine overall blood volume because the kidneys push water into the blood or withdraw water from the blood to bring the concentrations of these electrolytes within homeostatic ranges.

Blood volume is an important factor in circulation. For values above the optimum range, the greater the blood volume, the harder the heart must work to pump the blood, and the greater the fluid pressure in the arteries. For values below the optimum range, the less the blood volume, and the weaker the pressure filtration in the glomeruli (as well as the effects of inadequate circulation in all tissues and organs). However, the urinary system, when functioning properly, maintains blood chemistry (electrolyte concentration in the plasma), even if that requires putting some strain on other systems.

Hormonal mechanisms to control blood volume

The *renin-angiotensin system* (RAS) (also called the *renin-angiotensin-aldosterone system* [RAAS]) is called into action when the presence of toxins in the blood signals low blood pressure in the glomeruli. Specialized kidney cells secrete the enzyme *renin,* also called *angtiotensinogenase,* which sets off a series of reactions in different organ systems, eventually resulting in the production of the hormone *angiotensin II,* a powerful vasoconstrictor. Angiotensin II also stimulates the secretion of the hormone aldosterone from the adrenal cortex, which causes Na+ to be reabsorbed from the nephrons into the blood. Where salt goes, water follows. The movement of water into the blood increases blood volume, which, along with the vasoconstriction, raises blood pressure and enhances the effectiveness of the glomerular filtration.

The pituitary gland secretes ADH when the hypothalamus senses dehydration (from a lack of water consumption or a loss of water through sweating, diarrhea, or vomiting). Sodium is reabsorbed by the nephrons but not enough water follows, so ADH causes more water to be reabsorbed from the urine, which decreases the amount of urine and helps maintain normal blood volume and pressure.

Atrial natriuretic hormone (ANH) is a polypeptide hormone secreted by heart muscle cells in response to signals from sensory cells in the atria that blood volume is too high. ANH prevents the kidneys from secreting renin. In fact, the overall effect of ANH is to counter the effects of the RAS. ANH acts to reduce the water, sodium, and adipose (fat molecules) loads on the circulatory system, thereby reducing blood pressure.

Regulating blood pH

The homeostatic range for blood pH is narrow. The optimum value is around 7.4 (slightly alkaline). *Alkalosis* (increase in alkalinity) is life-threatening at 7.8. *Acidosis* (increased acidity) is life-threatening at 7.0.

Neutral pH is 7.0, the value for water.

Acids and, to a lesser extent, *alkalis* (bases) are products or byproducts of metabolic processes. The digestion of fats produces fatty acids. Capillary exchange acidifies the blood because the metabolic waste carbon dioxide is combined with water in the red blood cells, forming carbonic acid. Muscle activity produces lactic acid. Some acids are ingested in food and drink. The kidneys respond to changes in blood pH by excreting acidic or basic ions into the urine.

Your body has buffering processes in which the kidneys are involved. A *buffer* is a type of chemical that binds with either acid or base as needed to increase or decrease the solution pH. Buffers are made in cells and available in the blood.

Three mechanisms work together to maintain tight control over blood pH:

✔ Minor fluctuations in pH are evened out by the mild buffering effects of substances always present in the blood, such as the plasma proteins.

✔ When sensors in the kidneys detect that the blood is too acidic, they induce the breakdown of the amino acid glutamine, releasing ammonia, a basic substance, into the blood. When the ammonia arrives at the kidney, it's exchanged for Na+ in the urine and eliminated.

✔ By far the most important buffer for maintaining acid-base balance in the blood is the carbonic-acid-bicarbonate buffer. The body maintains the buffer by eliminating either the acid (carbonic acid) or the base (hydrogen carbonate ions). Carbonic acid concentration can be reduced within seconds through increasing respiration — the excretion of carbon dioxide through the lungs increases pH. Hydrogen carbonate ions must be eliminated through the kidneys, a process that takes hours.

Chapter 8

Making Babies: The Reproductive System

● ●

In This Chapter

▶ Understanding what the reproductive system does

▶ Getting the gametes together

▶ Looking at the male and female reproductive organs

▶ Responding to the body's changes during pregnancy

● ●

*L*ike all animals, humans have an instinctive knowledge of mating. However, only humans have a need to understand the processes of mating and reproduction. This chapter gives you information about the anatomy and physiology of reproduction. You're on your own for info about dating and mating rituals.

Surveying the Functions of the Reproductive System

The anatomy and physiology of the reproductive system is dedicated to supporting your role in continuing the human species (whether or not you choose to fulfill that role). Or to look at it another way, the reproductive system is dedicated to making sure your admirable characteristics are present in the next generation. Or to look at it from the "selfish-gene perspective," your reproductive system is the means by which some genes replicate themselves and fight on in the never-ending battle for continuing existence.

Following is an overview of what the reproductive system is responsible for:

✔ **Making gametes:** The *gametes* are made within the organs of the female and male reproductive systems. Also called the *sex cells,* gametes are of two kinds: The *ova* (singular, *ovum*) are the female gametes, and the *sperm* (singular, *sperm*) are the male gametes. Specialized cells generate the gametes in a cell-division process called *meiosis* (see the "Crossing over with meiosis" section, later in the chapter). At the cell level, the processes are essentially identical in female and male bodies. At the tissue, organ, system, and organism levels, the processes are very different. (We fill you in on the various processes throughout this chapter.)

✔ **Moving gametes into place:** However differently ova and sperm are made, if the reproductive system is to succeed in its purpose, one ovum and one sperm must make their way to the same place at the same time under the right conditions for them to fuse. Many of the reproductive system's tissues and organs chaperone the gametes from the place and time of their production to another place, where they're most likely to encounter their destiny.

✔ **Gestating and giving birth:** Only the female reproductive system has organs for gestating a fetus and giving birth. (See the "Pausing for Pregnancy" section, later in the chapter, for a detailed discussion of pregnancy.)

✔ **Nurturing the newborn:** The female reproductive system has tissues and organs specialized for nourishing the newborn for the first few months of life, until the baby is capable of digesting other food.

Making Gametes

The process of meiosis includes the sequence of cell-level events that result in the formation of sex cells (gametes) from somatic cells. Meiosis is the only cellular process in the human life cycle that produces *haploid* cells.

Somatic cells are *diploid,* meaning each cell nucleus contains two complete copies of the DNA that came into being in the zygote. Sex cells (gametes) are *haploid,* meaning each cell nucleus contains one copy of the DNA of the mother (somatic) cell. When two gametes fuse to form the zygote, each contributes its DNA to the new zygote, which is, therefore, diploid.

In the following sections, we expand on the process of meiosis and how female and male gametes are produced. We also touch on what causes these sex cells to create a male or female zygote.

Crossing over with meiosis

A cell divides by *mitosis* for purposes of asexual reproduction and for growth, development, replacement, and repair. A cell divides by *meiosis,* on the other hand, to produce gametes — that is, for purposes of sexual reproduction. The process of meiosis is similar in its mechanics to the process of mitosis, but the two have several key distinctions.

The most obvious difference is that meiosis has two parts, called *meiosis I* and *meiosis II.* Each part proceeds in a sequence of events similar to that of mitosis (prophase, metaphase, anaphase, and telophase). As we explain in Chapter 2, in mitosis, the mother cell is diploid, and both daughter cells are also diploid, each having one complete and identical copy of the mother cell's genome. In contrast, meiosis, when it functions optimally, results in four haploid daughter cells. What's more, the four haploid genomes are all different.

The early stages of meiosis include a mechanism called *crossing-over* or *recombination* for exchanging genes between chromosomes. The result is that the cell that becomes the gamete (one of the four haploid products of meiosis) is carrying chromosomes that are completely unique and not identical to the mother cell's chromosomes.

Note that replication of DNA *does occur* in meiosis, during the interphase that precedes the onset of meiosis I. After two sequential dichotomous divisions, the two complete copies are distributed among the four daughter cells.

Producing female gametes: Ova

A mature ovum (see Figure 8-1) is one of the largest cells in the human body, about 120 micrometers in diameter (about 25 times larger than sperm) and visible without magnification. The ovum contains a haploid nucleus, ample cytoplasm, and all the types of organelles usually found in the somatic cell, all within a plasma membrane. The plasma membrane is enclosed within a glycoprotein membrane called the *zona pellucida,* which protects the zygote and pre-embryo until implantation.

Oogenesis (the development of ova) in humans begins in embryonic and fetal development with specialized somatic cells called *oogonia*. A few of these cells head down the path of meiosis, producing cells called *primary oocytes*. However, this meiosis is suspended at the prophase I point until the female reaches puberty. At birth, the human female has about 700,000 oogonia and primary oocytes in suspended meiosis.

The primary oocyte undergoes meiosis I, producing two cells, called a *secondary oocyte* and the *first polar body*. Most of the primary oocyte's cytoplasm moves to the secondary oocyte. The first polar body undergoes meiosis II, and its daughter cells degenerate.

The cells released from the ovary at ovulation are secondary oocytes. If the secondary oocyte isn't fertilized, it degenerates without undergoing meiosis II.

When (or if) a sperm initiates fertilization, the secondary oocyte immediately undergoes meiosis II, producing the ovum (plus a second polar body, which degenerates). Following fertilization, the ovum contains the sperm nucleus, and after approximately 12 hours, the two haploid nuclei fuse, producing the zygote.

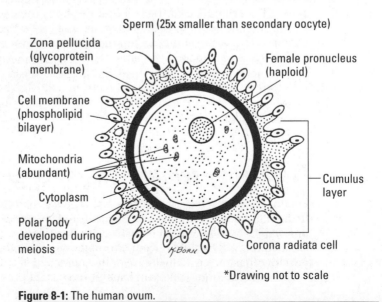

Sperm (25x smaller than secondary oocyte)

Zona pellucida (glycoprotein membrane)

Female pronucleus (haploid)

Cell membrane (phospholipid bilayer)

Mitochondria (abundant)

Cytoplasm

Polar body developed during meiosis

Cumulus layer

Corona radiata cell

K.BORN

*Drawing not to scale

Figure 8-1: The human ovum.

Developing male gametes: Sperm

A mature sperm has three parts: a head that measures about 5 x 3 micrometers, containing a haploid nucleus; a short middle section; and a long flagellum. The sperm is adapted for traveling light — it has very little cytoplasm. The head is covered by a structure that contains enzymes that break down the ovum's membrane to allow entry. The middle contains mitochondria and little else. Mitochondria produce the energy that fuels the sperm's highly active flagellum, which propels the sperm through the female reproductive tract.

The process of sperm development *(spermatogenesis)* from meiosis to maturation takes place inside the *testes.* Specialized cells called *spermatogonia* divide by mitosis to produce another generation of spermatogonia. Mature spermatogonia, called *primary spermatocytes,* divide by meiosis, producing four haploid gametes.

Similar to the case with females, males are born with spermatogonia in their *seminiferous tubules,* which remain dormant until puberty. During puberty, hormonal mechanisms pull the spermatogonia out of dormancy.

In contrast to oogenesis, which is cyclic, spermatogenesis is continuous beginning at puberty and continuing lifelong in some men. In contrast to the one-per-month gametogenesis in females, males produce astronomical numbers of sperm. Each ejaculation produces about 1 teaspoon of semen, which contains about 400 million sperm in a matrix of seminal fluid. Mature sperm can live in the epididymis and vas deferens for up to six weeks.

Merging ova and sperm to determine sex

An important difference between males and females is that in females, all chromosome pairs are made up of two identical-looking strands, whereas in males, the strands are different from each other. This difference is easily visible under a high-power microscope: One of the pair is "normal" length (about the same length as all the other chromosomes) and the other is markedly shorter than all other chromosomes. The first is called the X chromosome, and females have one set of them in all their somatic cells. The second is called the Y chromosome, and males have a mismatched pair (one X and one Y chromosome) in all their somatic cells. After meiosis in the female, all ova have one X chromosome. After meiosis in the male, each sperm has either an X or a Y. The fusion of an ovum with an X sperm produces a female (XX) zygote. The fusion of an ovum with a Y sperm produces a male (XY) zygote.

The Egg-citing Female Reproductive System

Among mammals, which include humans, the female body is specialized for reproduction to a much greater extent than the male body. The following sections introduce you to the various organs of the female reproductive system and walk you through the female menstrual cycle (which has to occur to prepare a woman's body for pregnancy).

A woman's reproductive organs

The organs of the female reproductive system are concentrated in the *pelvic cavity.* Many of the female reproductive organs are attached to the *broad ligament,* a sheet of tissue that supports the organs and connects the sides of the uterus to the walls and floor of the pelvis. The following sections go into detail about each of the woman's reproductive organs.

Ovaries

The *ovaries* are two almond-shaped structures approximately 2 inches (5 centimeters) wide, one on each side of the pelvic cavity. They house groups of cells called *follicles.*

The ovaries are the primary sex organs because they're the site of *oogenesis,* the process of oocyte maturation. The ovaries also have a major role in endocrine signaling, especially the production and control of hormones related to sex and reproduction.

Beginning at the female's puberty, the process of ovulation begins. The oogonia that have been dormant in her ovaries since early in her fetal development are hormonally activated, and secondary oocytes are released at a rate of approximately one per month from *menarche* (the first menstrual period) to *menopause* (the last menstrual period) — that is, from her early teen years to her late 40s or early 50s. The human female ovulates about 400 times during her lifetime.

Uterus

The *uterus*, or *womb*, nourishes and shelters the developing fetus during gestation. It's a muscular organ about the size and shape of an upside-down pear. The walls of the uterus are thick and capable of stretching as a fetus grows.

The lining of the uterus, called the *endometrium*, is built and broken down in the *menstrual cycle*, which we cover in the "A woman's (approximately) monthly cycle" section, later in the chapter. A portion of the endometrium *(deciduas basalis)* becomes part of the placenta during pregnancy.

The *uterine cervix* (neck) is a cylindrical muscular structure about 1 inch (2.5 centimeters) long that rests at the bottom of the uterus like a thimble. It controls the movement of biological fluids and other material (not to mention, occasionally, a baby) into and out of the uterus. Normally, the cervix is open ever so slightly to allow sperm to pass into the uterus. During childbirth, the cervix opens wide to allow the fetus to move out of the uterus.

Fallopian tubes

The *fallopian tubes* run from the ovary to the uterus. They're not connected to the ovaries; they just kind of hang over them. These tubes transport the released ovum to the uterus during the monthly cycle, or the *pre-embryo* (early-stage fetus) to the uterus in the event of conception.

Vagina

The *vagina* is the part of the female body that receives the male penis during sexual intercourse and serves as a passageway for sperm to enter into the uterus and fallopian tubes. The vagina is about 3 to 4 inches (8 to 10 centimeters) in length. The uterine cervix marks the top of the vagina.

During childbirth, the vagina must accommodate the passage of a fetus weighing, on average, about 7 pounds (3 kilograms), so the vagina's walls are made of stretchy tissues — some fibrous, some muscular, and some erectile. In their normal state, the vagina's walls have many folds, much like the stomach's lining.

When the vagina needs to stretch, the folds flatten out, providing more volume.

Vulva

In females, the external genitalia comprise the *labia majora, labia minora,* and the *clitoris.* Together, these organs are called the *vulva.* The term *labia* (singular, *labium*) means "lips." The labia of the vulva are loose flaps of flesh, just like the lips of the mouth. The labia protect the vagina's opening and cover the pelvis's bony structures.

Here are some details about the three parts of the vulva:

- ✔ **Labia majora:** These large folds of skin — one fold on each side — cover the smaller labia minora. The labia majora extend from the *mons pubis* (pubic mound) back toward the anus. The mons pubis contains fat deposits that cover the pubic bone. Following puberty, pubic hair covers the mons pubis and the labia majora.

- ✔ **Labia minora:** These hairless folds of skin lie underneath the labia majora and cover the opening of the vagina. The labia minora are attached near the vaginal opening and extend upward, forming the foreskin that covers the clitoris.

- ✔ **Clitoris:** This part of the vulva, located above the vagina's opening and above the urethra, has a shaft and glans tip, just as a penis does, and it's extremely sensitive to sexual stimulation. The clitoris contains erectile tissues that fill with blood during sexual stimulation. Because the tissue of the labia minora cap the clitoris, the swelling and reddening is also obvious in the labia minora. Stimulation of the clitoris can lead to orgasm in the female. Although females don't ejaculate, females do experience a building and release of muscular tension. Female orgasm causes the muscle tissue that lines the vagina and uterus to contract, which helps to pull the sperm up through the reproductive tract.

Breasts

Like other female mammals, female humans have mammary glands (breasts) that produce a substance called *milk* for the nutrition of relatively helpless infants with high calorie requirements. Besides nutrition, breast milk boosts the infant's immune system.

The breast contains about two dozen lobules that are filled with *alveoli* and contribute to ducts. The ducts merge at the *nipple*. Inside the alveoli are milk-producing cells. During puberty, the lobules and ducts form, and adipose tissue is deposited under the skin to protect the lobules and ducts and give shape to the breast. During pregnancy, hormones increase the number of milk-producing cells and increase the size of the lobules and ducts.

After the infant is born, the mother's pituitary gland secretes the hormone *prolactin,* which causes the milk-producing cells to create milk, and *lactation* begins. The infant suckles the milk out of the ducts through the nipple. Lactation continues as long as a child nurses regularly.

The hormone *oxytocin* is strongly involved in milk release (also known as the let-down reflex). Stimulation of the nipple prompts the secretion of oxytocin from the mother's pituitary gland. Oxytocin expels milk from the lobules by causing them to contract, just as it stimulates uterine contractions to expel the fetus. This hormone has also been strongly correlated with neuro-emotional phenomena, such as family bonding.

A woman's (approximately) monthly cycle

The *menstrual cycle (monthly cycle)* consists of the *ovarian cycle* and the *uterine cycle,* both of which are approximately 28 days in duration (see Figure 8-2). These cycles run concurrently to prepare the ovum and the uterus, respectively, for pregnancy.

By convention, the first day of menstrual bleeding is counted as Day 1 of the menstrual cycle. Menstrual bleeding begins at a point in the cycle when the levels of estrogen and progesterone are at their lowest. However, the entire menstrual cycle is directed by several hormones, not just estrogen and progesterone.

The next sections outline the phases of a woman's (monthly) menstrual cycle, up to menopause.

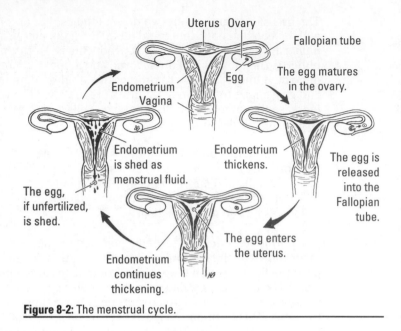

Uterus Ovary

Fallopian tube

The egg matures
in the ovary.

Egg

Endometrium
Vagina

Endometrium
is shed as
menstrual fluid.

Endometrium
thickens.

The egg is
released
into the
Fallopian
tube.

The egg,
if unfertilized,
is shed.

The egg enters
the uterus.

Endometrium
continues
thickening.

Figure 8-2: The menstrual cycle.

Looking at the ovarian cycle

The 28-day ovarian cycle is the most important part of the
menstrual cycle because it's responsible for producing the hormones that then control the uterine cycle (which we tell you
about in the next section). From Day 1 to Day 13, triggered by
low estrogen level, *follicle-stimulating hormone* (FSH) stimulates
the development of a follicle and *luteinizing hormone* (LH) stimulates the maturation of an oocyte in one of the ovaries. When
the follicle is developed enough, it begins to secrete estrogen.
When the level of estrogen reaches the appropriate level, a negative feedback mechanism involving the *hypothalamus* slows
the secretion of FSH and LH. When the follicle is fully mature
and the oocyte is ready to be released, FSH and LH secretion
peaks. On Day 14, the oocyte is released *(ovulation)*. An oocyte
lives for only 12 to 24 hours after ovulation.

At the time of ovulation, the anterior pituitary gland, which has
been secreting FSH and LH simultaneously, secretes a surge of
LH that causes the follicle from which the oocyte was released
to become a *corpus luteum* (yellow body). The corpus luteum
secretes the hormone *progesterone*, which triggers the hypothalamus. When the corpus luteum has secreted a sufficient
amount of progesterone, the hypothalamus stops the anterior

pituitary gland from secreting any more LH. At that point, the corpus luteum begins to shrink (about Day 17). When the corpus luteum is gone (about Day 26), the levels of estrogen and progesterone are at the lowest levels of the cycle (sometimes causing symptoms of premenstrual syndrome), and menstruation starts (about Day 29, or Day 1 of the new cycle).

Like any cycle, the whole process starts over. When the level of estrogen is low during menstruation, the hypothalamus detects the low level and secretes *gonadotropin-releasing hormone* (GnRH), which prompts the anterior pituitary gland to release its gonadotropic hormone — FSH — so another follicle is stimulated to develop a new oocyte that secretes estrogen. And now you're back to the first paragraph of this section.

Clocking the uterine cycle

The 28-day uterine cycle, which aims to prepare the uterus for a possible pregnancy, overlaps with the ovarian cycle.

- ✔ **Days 1 to 5:** The first 5 days of the uterine cycle is when the level of estrogen and progesterone are lowest — the period of menstruation. The low level of sex hormones fails to prevent the tissues lining the uterus (the *endometrium*) from disintegrating and shedding. As the hormone levels drop, blood vessels spasm, cells undergo *autolysis* (self-destruction), tissues tear apart from the uterine wall, and blood vessels rupture, causing the bleeding that occurs during a period. The blood and tissue (menstrual flow) passes out of the uterus through the cervix and then out of the body through the vagina.

- ✔ **Days 6 to 14:** During this *proliferative phase,* estrogen production is highest. The developed follicle secretes estrogen, which makes the endometrium regenerate fresh tissue. The tissues lining the uterus and the glands in the uterine wall grow and develop an increased supply of blood. All these changes are preparation for nourishing an embryo and supporting a pregnancy, should the oocyte, which is released on Day 14, become fertilized and implant in the wall of the uterus.

- ✔ **Days 15 to 28:** During this *secretory phase,* the corpus luteum secretes an increasing level of progesterone, which further thickens the endometrium, and the glands of the uterus secrete a thick mucus. If the egg becomes fertilized, the thickened endometrium and mucus help to "trap" the fertilized egg so it implants properly in the uterus. If the egg doesn't become fertilized within a day or two, the corpus luteum begins to shrink because it won't be needed for a pregnancy. As the corpus luteum shrinks, the progesterone and estrogen levels decline, which causes the endometrium to "shred and shed" just before menstruation.

Winding down the cycle

Physiologically, menopause essentially reverses the hormonal pathway of adolescence. When a woman enters menopause, her ability to reproduce ends — ovulation stops, and she no longer can become pregnant. She may also experience hot flashes and sweat baths if faulty signals from the parasympathetic nervous system disrupt the body's ability to accurately monitor its temperature. Other body processes slow down, including cellular metabolism and the replacement of the structural proteins in the skin, which leads to wrinkles. A woman's bones may also weaken when the breakdown of bone tissue occurs faster than the buildup of bone tissue during bone remodeling.

Menopause is one of the unique aspects of human physiology. Note that reproductive cycling declines and stops as the female ages. That happens in many mammal, bird, and reptile species (although relatively few individuals in any species live long enough to experience the decline of their reproductive capabilities).

The unique part is that human females often live a substantial proportion of their life span beyond their reproductive capacity. (A woman in her 80s has lived around 40 percent of her life after menopause.) Much research into this phenomenon is concentrated at the interface of biology and culture. One theory holds that an adult female with no offspring of her own to feed tends, instead, to feed her grandchildren or other children in her community. Children with grannies eat better, the theory goes, improving their chances of surviving to reproductive age and pushing her genes into one more generation.

Furthering Fertilization: The Male Reproductive System

The male reproductive system produces sperm and moves them into the female reproductive system. On a rare occasion (relative to the astronomical number of sperm that the average human male produces), a sperm fertilizes an egg. All the billions and billions of other sperm a man produces in his lifetime have a limited life span — about six weeks.

The female gamete is released from the ovary as a secondary oocyte. Only when fertilization is initiated does the ovum (egg) come into being.

A man's reproductive organs

The organs of the male reproductive system produce gametes, called sperm, and transfer them to the female reproductive system. In contrast to some other organ systems, and especially to the reproductive system of females, the male reproductive organs are located in an exposed location on the periphery of his body. The heart, lungs, kidneys, and the female's ovaries and uterus are all located beneath protective layers of skin, muscle, and other connective tissue and suspended in a fluid matrix, all of which support homeostasis in these organs. The exposed location of the male reproductive organs is common in mammals but unusual in other vertebrates.

Testes and scrotum

The *testes* (singular, *testis*) are paired organs that produce sperm and hormones. Like the ovaries of the female reproductive system, the testes are the site of gamete production and, therefore, the *primary sex organs*.

The testes contain fibrous tissue that forms compartments in the testis. Inside the compartments are long, coiled *seminiferous tubules*, the site of *spermatogenesis*, the process of sperm development from meiosis to maturation. The walls of the seminiferous tubules are lined with thousands of *spermatogonia* (immature sperm). The seminiferous tubules also contain *Sertoli cells* that nourish the developing sperm and regulate how many of the spermatogonia are developing at any one time.

The *epididymis* (plural, *epididymides*) is a long, cordlike structure that lies atop each testis. The epididymis is continuous with (that is, "becomes") the *vas deferens*, which is the final place of maturation for sperm. The vas deferens is a tube that connects the epididymis of each testis to the penis.

The testes are held within the *scrotum* beneath and outside of the abdomen. The scrotum contains smooth muscle that contracts when the scrotal skin senses cold temperatures and pulls the scrotum (and thereby the testicles) closer to the body to keep the sperm at the right temperature. The scrotum's inside muscle layers are an outpouching of the pelvic cavity. The scrotum's outside skin is continuous with the skin of the perineum and groin.

Prostate gland

Several other structures secrete the substances that make up the ejaculatory fluid that provides a matrix for the propulsion of sperm into the female reproductive tract. Among these are the *prostate* and the *seminal vesicles*. The prostate also contains some smooth muscles that help expel semen during ejaculation.

Penis

The penis consists of a shaft and the *glans penis* (tip). The tube-shaped *urethra* runs through the shaft of the penis, and the *glans penis* contains the *urethral orifice*. The semen is ejaculated through the urethra and urethral orifice. *Foreskin* (also called *prepuce*) covers the glans penis, although the foreskin of newborn males is often removed in a surgical procedure called *circumcision*.

During sexual arousal, erectile tissue enables the penis to be inserted into the female vagina, delivering the sperm to the vicinity of the secondary oocyte (if one is available).

Seminal fluid and ejaculation

The *seminal vesicles*, glands located at the juncture of the bladder and vas deferens, have ducts that allow the fluid they produce to sweep the sperm from the vas deferens into the urethra.

Next, the *prostate gland* adds its fluid, which contains mainly citric acid and a variety of enzymes that keep semen liquefied. The prostate gland surrounds the urethra just below where it exits from the urinary bladder.

The *bulbourethral glands*, also called *Cowper's glands*, sit within the floor of the pelvis near the bulb of the penis on either side of the urethra. These two small glands have ducts leading directly to the urethra.

These three types of glands — the seminal vesicles, the prostate gland, and the bulbourethral glands — secrete fluids that have several functions:

✓ They're slightly basic with a pH of 7.5, just the way sperm like their environment to be.

✓ They nourish the sperm by providing the sugar fructose so the sperm's mitochondria can make enough energy to move its tail and travel all the way to the egg.

✓ They contain *prostaglandins,* which are chemicals that make the uterus reverse its downward contractions. When the uterus contracts, the sperm are pulled farther upward into the female's reproductive tract.

As the glands add the secretions, forming the semen, pressure builds up on the structures of the male reproductive tract. When the pressure has reached its peak, the semen is expelled out of the urethra through the penis. Peristaltic waves and rhythmic contractions move the sperm through the vas deferens and urethra. The term for this discharge is *ejaculation* — part of orgasm in males, as is the contraction and relaxation of skeletal muscles at the base of the penis. As the muscles contract rhythmically, the semen comes out in spurts.

Pausing for Pregnancy

Pregnancy is established in two stages: fertilization of the secondary oocyte and implantation of the blastocyst in the uterus. The female body makes many and various adaptations to accommodate pregnancy and delivery, which we examine in the following sections.

Achieving fertilization

Ovulation sends a secondary oocyte from the follicle of the ovary into the uterine tube. Then, within an appropriate time, heterosexual intercourse results in the ejaculation of semen into the vagina. Some few million sperm make their way through the cervix, up through the uterus, and into the uterine tube to the vicinity of the waiting secondary oocyte.

To achieve fertilization, one sperm must penetrate the secondary oocyte's membrane, which initiates meiosis II, and its nucleus must fuse with that of the ovum. At this point, the secondary oocyte is fertilized, the ovum is developed, and, with the fusion of the nuclei, the zygote comes into being.

The probability of any act of intercourse resulting in fertilization is actually quite low because many complicating factors exist. The timing of intercourse relative to ovulation is crucial. The released secondary oocyte is viable for only a matter of hours; sperm live a little longer in the female reproductive tract (12 to 72 hours). The environment within the female reproductive tract may be more or less hospitable to the sperm, depending on the female's hormone levels and other physiological processes. Even when a single sperm has made contact with the secondary oocyte, fertilization is not assured.

Succeeding with implantation

Following fertilization, the zygote divides immediately. Several more cell division cycles take place as the pre-embryo moves down the uterine tube. Experts believe that many pre-embryos die at this stage, sometimes because of genetic or developmental abnormalities. Only if the pre-embryo arrives at the uterus and properly embeds itself into the endometrium is pregnancy established.

A successfully implanted pre-embryo, now called a *blastocyst,* begins immediately to take over its mother's body. It begins to produce a hormone called *human chorionic gonadotropin* (hCG), which maintains the *corpus luteum,* elevates levels of progesterone and estrogen, and inhibits menstruation.

Adapting to pregnancy

The maternal body responds to pregnancy with many anatomical and physiological changes to accommodate the growth and development of the fetus. Most structures and processes revert to the nonpregnant form (more or less) after the end of the pregnancy.

Uterus

During pregnancy, the uterus grows to about five times its nonpregnant size and weight to accommodate not only the

fetus but also the placenta, the umbilical cord, about a quart
of amniotic fluid, and the fetal membranes. The size of the
uterus usually reaches its peak at about 38 weeks gestation. During the last few weeks of pregnancy, the uterus has
expanded to fill the abdominal cavity all the way up to the
ribs. The size of the expanded uterus and the pressure of the
full-grown fetus may make things difficult for the mother.

The placenta acts as a temporary endocrine gland during
pregnancy, producing large amounts of estrogen and progesterone by 10 to 12 weeks. It serves to maintain the growth of
the uterus, helps to control uterine activity, and is responsible for many of the changes in the maternal body.

Near the end of pregnancy, the uterine cervix softens.
Enlarged and active mucus glands in the cervix produce the
operculum, a mucus "plug" that protects the fetus and fetal
membranes from infection. The mucus plug is expelled at the
end of the pregnancy. Additional changes and softening of the
cervix occur at the onset of labor.

Ovaries

Hormonal mechanisms prevent follicle development and
ovulation in the ovaries during pregnancy.

Breasts

The breasts usually increase in size as pregnancy progresses and
may feel inflamed or tender. The areolas of the nipples enlarge
and darken. The areola's *sebaceous glands* enlarge and tend to
protrude. By the 16th week (second trimester), the breasts begin
to produce *colostrum,* the precursor of breast milk.

Other organ systems

Pregnancy affects all organ systems as they support the
growth and development of the fetus and maintain homeostasis in the female. Here are a few important physiological consequences of pregnancy:

  ✔ The other abdominal organs are displaced to the sides
    as the uterus grows.

  ✔ Decreased tone and mobility of smooth muscles slows
    peristalsis and enhances the absorption of nutrients.
    An increase in water uptake from the large intestines
    increases the risk for constipation. Relaxation of the

cardiac sphincter may increase regurgitation and heart-burn. Nausea and other gastric discomforts are common.

✔ Increases occur in blood volume, cardiac output, body core temperature, respiration rate, urine volume, and output from sweat glands.

✔ Immunity is partially suppressed.

✔ Spinal curvature is realigned to counterbalance the growing uterus. Slight relaxation and increased mobility of the pelvic joints prepares the pelvis for the passage of the infant. This can compromise the woman's lower-body strength starting in the second trimester.

Going through labor and delivery

Labor is initiated by complex hormonal signaling between the maternal and fetal bodies. In the ideal labor and delivery process, powerful contractions of the smooth muscle of the uterus push the fully mature fetus (infant) past the cervix and down the birth canal without undue trauma to either the mother or the infant.

Labor occurs in three stages:

✔ **Stage 1** begins with regular, effective uterine contractions. The uterine cervix begins to *efface* (become thinner and wider), and the *amniotic membrane* ruptures.

✔ **Stage 2** involves continued uterine contractions pushing the fetus down through the birth canal. The cervix becomes fully effaced. The mother is aware of the passage of the fetus and may feel a strong urge to bear down and actively push the infant along.

At the *transition phase,* the infant emerges head first from the birth canal, marking the end of this stage of labor.

Just after delivery, the infant's umbilical cord is cut and tied off. The infant is now totally separated from the mother and will soon have a stylish belly-button.

✔ **Stage 3** starts after the baby is delivered. Uterine contractions continue so the placenta separates from the uterine wall. About 15 minutes after the baby is born, the placenta passes through the birth canal. Uterine contractions continue, during which the uterus contracts, eventually returning to near prepregnancy size.

Chapter 9

Exploring the Nervous, Endocrine, and Immune Systems

● ●

In This Chapter

▶ Linking the body's actions and reactions through the nervous system

▶ Surveying the glands and hormones that make up the endocrine system

▶ Protecting your body and fighting illness with the immune system

● ●

An organism's awareness of itself and of its environment depends on communication between one part of its body and another. In biology, such internal messaging is accomplished by several different mechanisms. Humans, like all mammals, use mechanisms involving chemistry and mechanisms involving electricity.

As we explore in this chapter, the nervous system is the body's electrical communications network. It generates and transmits information throughout the body by converting chemical signals into electrical impulses. The nervous system works closely with the endocrine system, which influences almost every cell, organ, and function of your body by releasing hormones from various glands. The nervous system controls when the endocrine system should release or withhold hormones.

In this chapter, we also consider the immune system. Your immune system is all that stands between you and a planet full of invasive microorganisms that regard you, metaphorically speaking, as a large serving of biological molecules that could feed their own processes.

Controlling It All: The Nervous System

The nervous system reaches into every organ and participates one way or another in nearly every physiological reaction. Perceiving the beauty of a flying bird and digesting your breakfast can happen simultaneously, and each action is dependent on the nervous system.

The nervous system has just three jobs to do, and these jobs overlap:

✓ **Sensory input:** Specialized neurons called *sensory receptors* collect information from the entire body, create an impulse, and transmit the impulse to either the spinal cord or brain stem, and then to the brain.

✓ **Integration:** The *central nervous system* (CNS) makes sense of the input it receives from all around the body.

✓ **Motor output:** In response to the integration of the sensory input, the *peripheral nervous system* (PNS) initiates and sends out impulses through nerves to muscles, glands, and other organs capable of the appropriate response.

The following sections get you acquainted with the various neural tissues and give you a glimpse at the inner workings of the CNS and PNS.

Surveying the neural tissues

The nervous system is made up primarily of two categories of cells — neurons and neuroglial cells — that associate very closely in the brain and in tissues called *nerves*.

Neurons

A *neuron* is an individual cell and is the basic unit of the nervous system. Neurons are highly specialized for the initiation and transmission of electrical signals (impulses). The neuron is able to, in an instant, receive the *outputs* (pulses of electrical energy) of many other cells, process this incoming information, and "decide" whether to generate its own signal to be passed on to other neurons, muscles, or gland cells.

Following are the three types of neurons (see Figure 9-1 for an illustration of the first two):

- ✔ **Sensory neurons:** Also called *afferent neurons* (*afferent* means "moving toward"), these neurons respond to sensory stimuli (touch, sound, light, and so on), passing the impulses ultimately to the spinal cord and brain.

- ✔ **Motor neurons:** Also called *efferent neurons* (*efferent* means "moving away"), these neurons transmit impulses from the brain and spinal cord to effector organs (muscles and glands), triggering responses from these organs (muscle contraction or release of the gland's product).

- ✔ **Interneurons:** Also called *association neurons,* these cells connect neurons to other neurons within the same region of the brain or spinal cord.

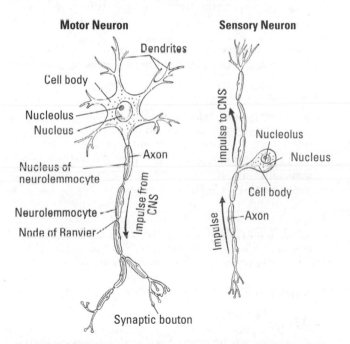

Figure 9-1: Motor neuron and sensory neuron, structure and path of impulses.

Neurons in different parts of the nervous system perform diverse functions and, therefore, vary in shape, size, and electrochemical properties. However, neurons have a special cellular anatomy adapted to the quick transmission of an electrical charge. All neurons have these same three parts, all enclosed within their cell membrane:

- ✔ **Cell body:** The body of a neuron is similar to a generic cell. It contains the nucleus, mitochondria, and other organelles.

- ✔ **Dendrites:** The dendrites are extensions that branch from one end of the cell body. They receive information from other neurons and send impulses in the direction of the cell body.

- ✔ **Axon:** The axon is a cable-like projection located on the opposite end of the cell body from the dendrite. Extending many times (tens, hundreds, or even tens of thousands of times) the cell body's diameter in length, the axon carries the impulses away from the cell body and toward the next neuron in the chain. (Think of electrical transmission wires.)

Fully differentiated neurons don't typically divide and may live for years, or even the whole lifetime of an organism.

Neuroglial cells

Various types of cells, collectively called *neuroglial cells* (or just *glial cells; glia* means "glue"), support neurons in various ways, including physically holding them in place and supplying them with nutrients. They protect neurons from pathogens and remove dead neurons. Certain types of glial cells generate *myelin,* a fatty substance that wraps around axons and provides electrical insulation that allows the axons to transmit action potentials much more rapidly and efficiently. Scientists estimate that in the human brain, the total number of glia roughly equals the number of neurons, although the proportions vary in different brain areas.

Nerves

A *nerve* is a bundle of peripheral axons. An individual axon plus its myelin sheath is called a *nerve fiber.* Nerves provide a common pathway for the electrochemical nerve impulses that are transmitted along each of the axons. Nerves are found only in the PNS. Nerve fibers can be of two types: *motor,* which send impulses away from the CNS, or *sensory,* which send impulses toward the CNS.

Ganglia and plexuses

A *ganglion* (plural, *ganglia*) is literally a bundle of nerves. Well, almost literally. A ganglion is an aggregation of neuron cell bodies. Ganglia provide relay points and intermediary connections among the body's neurological structures, especially between the CNS and the PNS.

Ganglia may be connected to form a *chain*. For example, the sympathetic nervous system contains a chain of ganglia referred to as the *paravertebral ganglia* or the *sympathetic chain of ganglia*.

Plexus is a general term for a network of anatomical structures, such as lymphatic vessels, nerves, or veins. (The term comes from the Latin *plectere* meaning "to braid.") A neural plexus is a network of intersecting nerves. The *solar plexus* serves the internal organs. The *cervical plexus* serves the head, neck, and shoulders. The *brachial plexus* serves the chest, shoulders, arms, and hands. The *lumbar, sacral,* and *coccygeal plexuses* serve the lower body.

Traveling the integrated networks

The nervous system comprises two physically separate but functionally integrated networks of nervous tissue. Working together, these networks perceive and respond to internal and external stimuli to maintain homeostasis and simultaneously move the genetic development program forward. The following sections take a closer look at the central and peripheral nervous systems.

Central nervous system

The *central nervous system* (CNS), which consists of the brain and spinal cord, is the largest part of the nervous system. It integrates the information it receives from the sensory receptors and coordinates the activity of all parts of the body.

Both the brain and spinal cord are masses of neural tissue protected within bony structures (the skull and the vertebral column, respectively) and layers of membranes and specialized fluids, reflecting their prime importance to the continuation of the organism's life.

The brain and spinal cord are made up mainly of two types of tissue, called *gray matter* and *white matter*. Gray matter consists of unmyelinated neurons, neuron cell bodies, and neuroglial cells. White matter is made up of neuroglial cells and the myelinated axons extending from the neuron cell bodies in the gray matter. (See the "Surveying the neural tissues" section, earlier in this chapter, for more on neurons and neuroglial cells.) The myelin has a high fat content, which results in white matter's white color.

In the brain, the gray matter forms a thin layer on the outside (the *cortex*). The white matter is beneath and makes up the brain's big data lines, carrying information around the brain. In the spinal cord, the tissue is arranged in a long cylinder; the gray matter forms the inner layer, and the white matter forms the outer layer.

The spinal cord extends from the bottom of the brain stem down the vertebral column within a cylindrical tubular opening created by the vertebrae and three tough membranes with cushioning fluid between them.

Peripheral nervous system

The *peripheral nervous system* (PNS) consists of the nerves and ganglia outside of the brain and spinal cord. Unlike the CNS, the PNS isn't protected by bone or by the blood-brain barrier, leaving it exposed to toxins and mechanical injuries. Structures of the PNS include the following:

- **Cranial nerves:** Twelve pairs of nerves that emerge directly from the brain and brain stem. Each pair is dedicated to particular functions — some bring information from the sense organs to the brain, others control muscles, but most have both sensory and motor functions. Some are connected to glands or internal organs such as the heart and lungs. For example, the longest of the cranial nerves, called the *vagus nerves,* pass through the neck and chest into the abdomen. They relay sensory impulses from part of the ear, tongue, larynx, and pharynx; relay motor impulses to the vocal cords; and relay motor and secretory impulses to some abdominal and thoracic organs.

- **Spinal nerves:** Thirty-one pairs of nerves that emerge from the spinal cord. Each contains thousands of *afferent* (sensory) and *efferent* (motor) fibers.

✔ **Sensory nerve fibers:** Nerve fibers all over the body that send impulses to the CNS via the cranial nerves and spinal nerves.

✔ **Motor nerve fibers:** Nerve fibers that connect to muscles and glands and send impulses from the CNS via the cranial and spinal nerves.

REMEMBER

The PNS is further divided into the somatic system and the autonomic system.

✔ The *somatic nervous system* regulates activities that are under conscious control. Its sensory fibers receive impulses from receptors. Its motor fibers transmit impulses from the CNS to the (voluntary) skeletal muscles to coordinate body movements.

✔ The motor fibers of the *autonomic system* transmit impulses from the CNS to the glands, heart, and smooth (involuntary) organ muscles. The autonomic system controls internal organ functions that are involuntary and that happen subconsciously, such as breathing, heartbeat, and digestion. This system is made up of the following:

• **Sympathetic nervous system:** Nerves originate in the thoracic and lumbar regions of the spinal cord. The sympathetic nervous system responds to stress and is responsible for the increase of your heartbeat and blood pressure, among other physiological changes, along with the sense of excitement you may feel due to the increase of adrenaline in your system.

• **Parasympathetic nervous system:** Nerves originate in the brain stem and sacral portion of the spinal cord. The parasympathetic nervous system is evident when you rest or feel relaxed and is responsible for such things as the constriction of the pupil, the slowing of the heart, the dilation of the blood vessels, and the stimulation of the digestive and urinary systems. The parasympathetic nervous system is known as the *housekeeping* system because it maintains your normal functioning when you're not under stress.

• **Enteric nervous system:** This system manages every aspect of digestion, from the esophagus to the stomach to the small intestine to the colon.

Sending Messages Chemical-Style with the Endocrine System

In general, the endocrine system is in charge of body processes that happen slowly, such as cell growth. The nervous system, described in the earlier section "Controlling It All: The Nervous System,w" manages faster processes such as breathing and body movement. The following sections explain the functions of hormones and the glands they come from.

Homing in on hormones

A *hormone* is an *endogenous substance* (one that's produced within the body) that has its effects in specific target cells. Hormones are many and varied in their source, chemical nature, target tissues, and effects. However, they're characterized by the fact that they're synthesized in one place (gland or cell) and they travel via the blood until they reach their target cell. Hormones are bound by specific receptors in their target cells. The binding of the hormone on the receptor induces a response within the cell.

Among glands, the pituitary, thyroid, and adrenal glands are most well-known. These organs have no significant function other than to produce hormones. However, a number of other endocrine tissues and hormones, though less well-known, are just as important in controlling vital bodily functions. In fact, all the tissue in your body is, in some way, an endocrine tissue.

Hormone chemistry

Chemically, hormones fall into four types:

- ✔ **Lipid hormones:** Lipid and phospholipid hormones are derived from fatty acids. The best-known lipid hormones are the steroids, such as estrogen, progesterone, testosterone, aldosterone, and cortisol (which is synthesized from cholesterol). Another group of lipid hormones is called *prostaglandins*.

- ✔ **Peptide hormones:** Peptides are relatively short chains of amino acids. Peptide hormones include antidiuretic hormone (ADH), thyrotropin-releasing hormone (TRH), and oxytocin.

Other hormones are *proteins* (chains of peptides), such as insulin, growth hormone, and prolactin.

✓ **Glycoprotein hormones:** More complex protein hormones bear carbohydrate side-chains and are called *glycoprotein hormones*. These include follicle-stimulating hormone (FSH), luteinizing hormone (LH), and thyroid-stimulating hormone (TSH).

✓ **Amine hormones:** Amine hormones are derivatives of the amino acids tyrosine and tryptophan. Examples are thyroxine, epinephrine, and norepinephrine.

Hormone sources

At one time, and not so long ago, by definition a hormone was produced in an endocrine gland (and an endocrine gland was a structure that produced one or more hormones). But as biologists have discovered and described more and more hormone substances and forms, they've expanded the definition to include similar, sometimes identical, substances that have a similar mechanism of action, wherever they're produced. Check out all the sources of hormones:

✓ **Endocrine glands:** An *endocrine gland* is an organ that synthesizes a hormone. It does so within a specialized cell type — the anterior pituitary gland, for instance, has cells that specialize in the production of such hormones as adrenocorticotropic hormone (ACTH), growth hormone, and TSH. Specialized cells within the thymus synthesize hormones that control the maturation of immune cells.

✓ **Various organs:** A number of organs not usually included within the endocrine system by anatomists and physiologists have cells and tissues specialized for the production of hormones. For example:

  • While part of the pancreas is busy secreting enzymes for the digestion of food, other specialized cells of the pancreas produce insulin, and others produce glucagon.

  • The stomach and intestines, too, synthesize and release hormones that control both physical and chemical aspects of digestion.

  • Specialized cells in the ovaries and testes transform cholesterol molecules into molecules of estrogen and testosterone, respectively.

- Even the heart produces hormones, the secretion of which has an immediate strong effect on blood volume (fluid balance).

✔ **Neurons:** Neurons make hormones that are neurotransmitters. Or, to look at it another way, hormones are substances that transmit physiologically significant messages with considerable subtlety; therefore, not surprisingly, they're synthesized and released in different physiological messaging contexts — the transmission of nerve impulses across a synapse, for example. The only difference between epinephrine synthesized in the adrenal glands and epinephrine synthesized in nerve cells is the distance the molecules travel to their target site.

Hormone receptors

Hormones exit their cell of origin via *exocytosis,* which involves a sac or vesicle enveloping the substance and moving it across the cell membrane, or another means of membrane transport. A secreted hormone molecule goes directly into the blood and circulates until it enters a cell or binds with its specific receptor on the cell membrane, where through second messengers its effects may be profound.

The presence of a specific hormone receptor makes that cell a target for the hormone. Without the target receptor, the hormone has no effect.

The receptor may be *on* or embedded *in* the cell membrane, as is typically the case for peptide hormones. The hormone molecule, called the *first messenger,* is taken into the cell via active transport, stimulating the production of a compound, *cyclic AMP (cyclic adenosine monophosphate),* called the *second messenger,* thus causing the target cell to produce the necessary enzymes — that is, to induce the expression of a certain gene. (We describe the process of active transport in Chapter 2.)

A steroid hormone molecule doesn't require a cell-membrane receptor or active transport. As a lipid, it enters a cell by diffusing through the membrane. After it's inside the cell, it binds with target receptor molecules in the cytoplasm. The receptor-hormone complex moves into the nucleus, where it activates the expression of the gene for a needed enzyme.

Grouping the glands

In general, a *gland* is a structure that synthesizes a product that's exported from the cells. *Endocrine* (ductless) glands export their products (hormones) via the bloodstream to their target cells in anatomically distant organs. The following sections give you the lowdown on the endocrine glands.

The taskmasters: The hypothalamus and pituitary

The *hypothalamus* can be considered the location where the nervous system and the endocrine system meet. It's sometimes called the *master gland* because it ultimately controls the functioning of other glands, acting through the *pituitary*.

The hypothalamus contains special cells that act as sensors that "analyze" the composition of the blood as it circulates through. It also contains other specialized cells that generate messengers (hormones) in response to the analysis. Tight pairing between these two types of cells is essential for homeostasis.

The pituitary gland has two parts, called the *anterior pituitary* and *posterior pituitary,* that have different relationships with the hypothalamus.

- The anterior pituitary gland secretes many hormones, including melanocyte-stimulating hormone (MSH). This hormone directly stimulates melanocytes to produce melanin pigment, which protects the skin from sunlight damage. This gland also secretes *prolactin,* which is responsible for the increase in size of the lactiferous glands in the breast and the production of milk. It also secretes the gonadotropic hormones FSH and LH, which target the ovaries and testicles, and ACTH, which targets the cortex of the adrenal glands. The function of these pituitary hormones is to stimulate the release of other hormones from their target glands.

- The posterior pituitary gland, which is directly connected to the hypothalamus, releases hormones that are actually synthesized in the nerve cell bodies of the hypothalamus and travel down the axons that end in the posterior pituitary. One such hormone is ADH. When the blood's fluid volume falls below the ideal range, the hypothalamus produces ADH, which travels down the axons into the posterior pituitary gland. Released by the pituitary into the blood, ADH reaches its target kidney cells. Via active transport, ADH enters the cells of the tubules and alters the cells' metabolism so more water is removed from the urine that the kidney produces and is added to the blood.

Controlling metabolism

Two relatively small organs exert a major effect on the availability of energy for physiological processes:

✔ **The thyroid gland:** Straddling your *trachea* (windpipe) and looking somewhat like a butterfly, your thyroid gland secretes hormones that affect almost every physiological process in the body. The thyroid hormones

- Regulate the rate at which cells metabolize and respire (use oxygen and release carbon dioxide).

- Increase the rate at which cells use glucose and stimulate the breakdown of glycogen (the storage form of glucose) into individual glucose molecules so the blood level of glucose increases.

- Help maintain body temperature by increasing or decreasing metabolic rate.

- Regulate growth and differentiation of tissues in children and teens.

- Increase the amount of certain enzymes in the mitochondria that are involved in oxidative reactions.

- Influence the metabolic rate of proteins, fats, carbohydrates, vitamins, minerals, and water.

- Stimulate mental processes.

✔ **The adrenal gland:** Found near the kidneys, each adrenal gland consists of two parts, the *cortex* and the *medulla.*

- The adrenal cortex secretes *corticosteroids,* which include *mineralocorticoids, glucocorticoids,* and *gonadocorticoids.* One of the most important mineralocorticoids is *aldosterone,* which is responsible for regulating the concentration of *electrolytes,* such as potassium (K+), sodium (Na+), and chloride (Cl–) ions. This regulation keeps the blood's salt and mineral content within the ranges required for homeostasis. The main glucocorticoid hormone, *cortisol,* regulates the metabolism of proteins, fats, and carbohydrates. Your body releases cortisol when you're stressed emotionally, physically, or environmentally.

- The adrenal medulla, which developed from the same tissues as the sympathetic nervous system, is responsible for regulating a class of hormones called the *catecholamines,* of which *epinephrine* and *norepinephrine* are the best known. Epinephrine, also called *adrenaline,* initiates the adrenaline rush of the *fight-or-flight response.*

Getting the gonads going

Your *gonads* — *ovaries* if you're female or *testes* if you're male — produce and secrete the steroid sex hormones throughout your lifetime at different levels. Their production increases at puberty and normally decreases as you age. Here's the scoop on the different sex hormones:

- ✓ **Estrogen:** In women, the increased production of estrogen at puberty is responsible for initiating the development of the secondary sex characteristics, such as the enlargement of the breasts.

- ✓ **Progesterone:** This hormone works to prepare the uterus for implantation of a pre-embryo by causing changes in uterine secretions and in storing nutrients in the uterus's lining. Progesterone also contributes to breast development.

- ✓ **Testosterone:** This hormone causes the development of secondary sex characteristics in males.

Defending Your "Self" with the Immune System

Your *immune system* consists of a variety of components: the *lymphatic system,* a body-wide network of vessels and organs through which flows an important body fluid called *lymph;* a variety of very peculiar cell types; and several types of biological molecules, some of them just as peculiar. These components all have specialized functions for attacking and eliminating microbial invaders:

- ✓ **Confronting marauders:** Whether you're well or ill, your immune system is always alert and active. That's why none of the bacteria, fungi, parasites, and viruses that are present by the uncountable millions in the air you breathe, on surfaces you touch, and on your food, are eating you.

✔ **Stopping renegades:** The second major function of the immune system is to recognize and destroy cells of your own body that have gone rogue — potential seeds for cancerous growth.

Loving Your Lymphatic System

The *lymphatic system* plays a crucial role in circulation by draining the fluids that pour out into the extracellular space during capillary exchange and returning them to the blood. The lymphatic system is more than a drainage network, though. It removes toxins, helps transport fats, and stabilizes blood volume despite environmental stresses. Possibly its most interesting functions are those related to its role in the immune system, fighting biological invaders.

Lymphing along

Interstitial (extracellular) fluid is a watery solution containing oxygen, ions, glucose and other nutrients, proteins, hormones, and so on. The total volume of interstitial fluid, which is found in between cells, is about 2 to 4 pints (1 to 2 liters) at any given moment.

Like plasma, interstitial fluid is continuously flowing: The pressure of the heartbeat pushes this watery solution across the capillary cell membrane and out into the interstitial space, a total of about 50 pints (24 liters) per day. Most of it is reabsorbed into the blood at the venous end of the capillaries. The rest goes on a detour through the lymphatic system. The fluid coursing through the lymphatic system is called *lymph*. After passing through the lymphatic system, the fluid rejoins the circulatory system through two large veins and becomes plasma again.

Structures of the lymphatic system

The structures of the lymphatic system resemble those of other organs and systems that function to move fluids around. The lymphatic system has its own tubes, pipes, connectors, reservoirs, and filters. It lacks its own pumping organ but, like venous circulation, makes use of skeletal muscle action for this purpose.

Lymphatic vessels

The *lymphatic vessels* are the tubes that carry lymph. They form a network very similar to the venous system. You can even think of the lymphatic system as an alternative venous system, because the lymph that the vessels transport comes out of the arterial blood and is delivered back into the venous blood. Like the venous system, the lymphatic system's vessels start small (the lymph capillaries) and get larger (the lymphatic vessels), and even larger (the lymphatic ducts). Like veins, lymphatic vessels rely on skeletal muscle action and valves to keep the fluid moving in the right direction. The structure of the lymphatic vessel wall is similar to that of the veins, but thinner. Lymph vessels are distributed through the body, more or less alongside the blood vessels.

Lymphatic ducts

The largest of the lymphatic vessels, the *lymphatic ducts,* drain into two large veins. The right lymphatic duct, located on the right side of your neck near your right clavicle, drains lymph from the right arm and the right half of the body above the diaphragm into the *right subclavian vein.* The *thoracic duct,* also called the *left lymphatic duct,* which runs through the middle of your thorax, drains lymph from everywhere else into the *left subclavian vein.*

Lymph nodes

Lymph nodes are bean-shaped structures located along the lymph vessels. Dense clusters of lymph nodes are found in the mouth, pharynx, armpit, groin, all through the digestive system, and other locations. Each lymph node is covered by a fibrous connective tissue *capsule. Afferent* lymphatic vessels cross the capsule on the convex side, bringing lymph into the node. The node's *efferent vessel,* which carries the filtered lymph out of the node, emerges from the indentation on the concave side of the capsule, called the *hilus* (as in the kidney).

On the inner side, the capsule sends numerous extensions that divide the node internally into structures called *nodules.* A nodule is filled with a meshlike network of fibers to which *lymphocytes* and *macrophages* (another immune system cell type) adhere. As the lymph flows through the node, pathogens, cancerous cells, and other matter in the lymph are engulfed and destroyed by macrophages or marked for destruction by B lymphocytes. The cleaned-up lymph travels toward the venous system in the efferent vessels.

The lymph nodes also provide a safe and nurturing environ-ment for developing lymphocytes. (See the "Lymphocytes" section, later in the chapter.)

The splendid spleen

The *spleen* is a solid organ, located to the left of and slightly posterior to the stomach. It's roughly oval in shape, normally measuring about 1 x 3 x 5 inches (3 x 8 x 13 centimeters) and weighing about 8 ounces (23 grams). Essentially, its structure is that of a really large lymph node, and it filters blood in much the same way the lymph nodes filter lymph, removing pathogen cells along with exhausted RBCs and many kinds of foreign matter.

The spleen's structure is similar to that of other organs, like the kidney, the liver, and the lymph nodes. The spleen is enveloped by a fibrous capsule. The spleen has a *hilus,* a spot where several different vessels cross the capsule. The spleen's hilus contains the *splenic artery, the splenic vein,* and an *efferent lymph vessel,* a similar configuration to the lymph node. Note that the spleen has no role in filtering lymph and no afferent lymph vessels.

Inside, the spleen is divided into functional subunits by out-growths of the capsule's fibrous tissue. Within each subunit, an arteriole is surrounded by material called *white pulp* — lymphoid tissue that contains lymphocyte production cen-ters. Farther toward the outer edges of each compartment, similar masses called *red pulp* surround the arteriole. The red pulp is a network of channels filled with blood, where most of the filtration occurs. (It's also the major site of destruction of deteriorating RBCs and the recycling of their hemoglobin.) Both white pulp and red pulp contain *leukocytes* that remove foreign material and initiate an antibody-producing process.

The thymus gland

The *thymus gland* overlies the heart and straddles the trachea, sitting just posterior to the sternum. It produces *thymosin,* a hormone that stimulates the differentiation and matura-tion of T cells. The thymus is relatively large in childhood; it decreases in size with age.

Identifying immune system cells

Immune system cells are special in many ways. In shape and size, they're far from the compact epithelial or muscle cell types. Immune system cells have about a dozen distinctive shapes and many different sizes, and some have the ability to transform themselves into other, even weirder forms and to multiply extremely rapidly. The next sections give you a closer look at specific types of immune system cells.

Looking at leukocytes

Immune system cells are called *leukocytes* (white cells), because they appear white in color under a microscope. (That's *white* as in *pus*.) Although all blood cells, red and white, develop from *hematopoietic stem cells* in the red marrow, the leukocytes contain no hemoglobin and no iron. Unlike RBCs, all leukocytes retain their nuclei, organelles, and cytoplasm through their life cycle. Many fewer leukocytes are produced than RBCs, by a factor of around 700.

Also called *white blood cells* (WBCs), leukocytes are present everywhere and function at all times. You notice their presence in the acute phase of certain diseases — the immune response, not the invader directly, produces the well-known symptoms of flu. They function not only in the blood (really, in the plasma) but also in the interstitial fluid and the lymph. They're never far from a site of injury or infection because they're everywhere. When a splinter pierces your finger, a contingent of local WBCs arrives at the site instantaneously.

Sometimes it's difficult to remember that these bizarre warrior cells with their amazing superpowers are your cells, just like your skin cells and your blood cells. Discussing them is difficult without resorting to language that makes them seem like a quasi-military force from outside your body. These cells are acutely aware (metaphorically speaking) that "they" are "self" (you). In fact, that's the primary distinction that matters to them: *self* or *nonself*. The overarching mission of a leukocyte is to protect self from other *biotic* (living) nonself, destroying the invaders where possible and necessary and establishing more or less mutualistic relationships with other life forms where possible and necessary. It's hard not to picture a disciplined army; but remember it's a metaphor.

Lymphocytes

The *lymphocytes* are one group of leukocytes (WBCs). The group includes the B cells and T cells (small, agranular lymphocytes), as well as NK cells (large granular lymphocytes). To simplify: Activated B cells produce antibodies; some T cells destroy antigens; and NK cells attack cancerous cells and cells infected by viruses. The surfaces of lymphocytes are covered with receptors, which are molecules that fit with a specific *antigen*.

All lymphocytes originate in the red marrow from the same type of hematopoietic stem cell. B lymphocytes and NK cells leave the marrow fully differentiated and enter the circulatory and lymphatic systems. T cells travel to the thymus gland to complete their differentiation in an environment rich in the hormone *thymosin*. Then they move to the medulla of a lymph node, where they further differentiate into one of several different cell types, each with its own function in the immune response: helper T cells, *cytotoxic* (cell killing) T cells, or suppressor T cells.

Phagocytizing leukocytes

Several different types of WBCs perform their function in part by processes involving *phagocytosis* (the digestion of foreign material).

- *Neutrophils* are the most numerous of the WBCs (40 to 70 percent of the total number) and are continuously present and active in the circulatory and lymphatic systems. Neutrophils squeeze through the capillary walls and into infected tissue, where they phagocytize the invading bacteria. They also function to limit the populations of the beneficial bacterial species in the respiratory and digestive passages.

- *Monocytes* aren't really stem cells, but they have some functions in common with stem cells — they exist to produce other specialized cells on demand. Monocytes divide to produce two other kinds of immune cells, *macrophages* and *dendritic cells*. In a homeostatic state, the monocytes replenish these cells as necessary. In response to inflammation-response-related stimuli, monocytes travel to the site and begin to turn out vast numbers of its daughter cells.

  Macrophages (literally, "big eaters") are large phagocytic cells that target antigens and dead self cells. In the early stages of the immune response, macrophages initiate the mass production of other types of WBCs. Dendritic cells take macrophagy to a whole new level beyond the scope of this book.

Chapter 10

Ten Phabulous Physiology Phacts

. . . .

In This Chapter

▶ Ruminating on your thumbs, hair, nose, and mouth

▶ Making friends with microbes and milk

▶ Taking in oxygen and transporting it with hemoglobin

. . . .

This merest smattering of the everyday miracles of the anatomy and physiology of human beings inspires awe at the power of evolution's forces.

Only Humans Have Opposable Thumbs

One specialization that differentiates humans from other animals is the *opposable thumb*, which is a thumb that can touch each finger on the same hand. (Go ahead — try it now.) Along with that, the human thumb is *prehensile*, meaning capable of grasping. This anatomy underlies the development of manual dexterity and fine motor skills in humans. The prehensile, opposable thumb makes possible tool making, hunting and gathering, textile and metal crafts, art, writing, cooking, and possibly the very existence of human culture.

Human Milk Is the Best Milk

The best nutrition for a human baby is human milk. Human milk is a complex mixture of more than 200 different components, and no other substance produced in another animal, or yet in a laboratory, matches its ability to meet the needs of a human infant.

Like all foods, the core components of milk are carbohydrates, proteins, and fats. Human milk also contains many other substances that affect nutrition and development in different ways. Milk and its precursor, *colostrum,* essentially lend the baby part of the mother's immune system until it can make its own: B cells, T cells, neutrophils, macrophages, and antibodies. Milk also has human hormones and growth factors that are believed by some to be required to optimize the development of the brain and other organs.

You're (Surprisingly) as Hairy as a Gorilla

Among the great apes, the genus Homo is distinguished by an apparent lack of hair. Evolutionary theorists suggest that the ape forebears of Homo were about as hairy as gorillas, who put their hair to many uses, including mechanical protection, UV protection, thermoregulation, sexual selection, social signaling, and waterproofing.

Anatomists note that humans haven't "lost" their hair — the skin is covered with hair follicles at about the same density as other apes. But the hair itself is different. Most of it is short and fine. Head hair is longer and coarser than body hair. Head hair and body hair may be curly. (No other ape has curly hair anywhere.) It may be lightly pigmented or apigmented. How does Homo escape a predator or thermoregulate under that? Maybe he runs away on his long, hairless legs, cooled by a steady stream of water from newly evolved glands on his hairless chest and arms. Homo evolved evaporative cooling for a hunter's life on the hot, dry, equatorial savannah.

You Can Process Fear and Emotion

The *amygdalae* are paired structures in the middle brain almost exactly the size and shape of almonds, which is where they get their name. The amygdalae have been associated clinically with a range of mental and emotional conditions, including religious rapture, depression, autism, and even "normalcy."

Physicians have widely and publicly discussed one case in particular — a woman whose amygdalae are partly nonfunctional. This patient is incapable of experiencing the emotion of fear. The doctors have tried everything, not just for research purposes but because a total lack of fear is a maladaptive trait; it threatens her well-being and survival. This patient has been injured and victimized in situations that normal, healthy fear would have kept her far away from.

You Smell Like You See

As with other mammals, the human olfactory structures are located at the interface of the brain and the airway. Specialized neurons called *olfactory neurons*, actually protuberances from the brain, sit right on the border of the nasal passages, behind and slightly above the nostrils. An olfactory neuron bears olfactory receptors on its plasma membrane. An olfactory receptor recognizes a certain chemical feature of an odor molecule, but that feature is present in numerous kinds of odor molecules. The receptor can bind any odor molecules that have that feature. Thus, humans don't have a single receptor for "coffee" or "lavender" or "wet dog." They have many receptors for many kinds of molecules released into the air and drawn into the nose. The brain assembles its olfactory perception of the environment by aggregating the signals from the various receptors. The process is similar to that of vision. Odor recognition is like object recognition based on aggregating many different impulses from the retina.

Your Mouth Is More Efficient Than a Chimp's

Compared with other apes, the human *buccal* apparatus (mouth) is puny. The capacity of the male adult human mouth is about the same as that of the male adult chimp, who is only about two-thirds the man's size. The chimp can open twice as wide, showing teeth about twice as big. The man has nothing like the chimp's enormous, muscular lips for expressing juice from fibrous foods. The human *temporalis* and *masseter* muscles are small and weak compared with the chimp's powerful jaw muscles. Yet, with all this extra power, the chimp spends about six hours each day masticating (chewing food), whereas the human hunter-gatherer spends less than one hour. Yes, the puny mouth of a human chews food much more effectively than the mighty mouth of a chimp.

Millions of Microbes Owe You Their Lives

For thousands of millions of tiny creatures, your gut is the only universe they know. They live and die in that warm, moist, nutrient-rich, immune-protected environment. They work almost every minute of their lives, providing a service to their community and their universe. These good citizens of the gut are adapted specifically to that environment, in the way of symbiotic organisms, and can survive nowhere else.

The internal tissues — blood, bone, muscle, and the others — are normally free of microbes. But the surface tissues — the skin, the digestive and respiratory tracts, and the female urogenital tract — have distinctive colonies of symbiotic microorganisms. The term *symbiosis* (adjectival form, *symbiotic*) describes a more or less cooperative and reciprocal relationship between organisms and species.

Oxygen Can be Dangerous

It was the biggest environmental disaster ever on the planet. After life forms had gotten along for a billion years or so, obtaining energy from chemosynthetic processes, some bacterial forms evolved the ability to capture the energy of light itself. This was a huge advantage for them, but unfortunately for all life forms then in existence, photosynthesis has a toxic byproduct: molecular oxygen. Slowly, as photosynthesizing bacteria prospered, overly reactive molecular oxygen replaced moderately reactive methane in the earth's atmosphere.

We can only speculate about what happened next, and some cell biologists have speculated very imaginatively. They started by noticing the strong similarities between certain organelles and some bacteria (between mitochondria and rod-shaped bacteria, for example). Then came the stunning discovery that mitochondria and *chloroplasts* (the photosynthesizing organelles of plant cells) had their own DNA, completely separate from the genomic DNA in the nucleus, and that this DNA was bacterial in character. Gradually, the view has come to be accepted that eukaryotic cells began as symbiotic communities of different types of bacteria sheltering from the damaging effects of atmospheric oxygen inside a bubble of phospholipid bilayer.

You Can Control Your Breathing but Fido Can't

You don't have to think about breathing. The steady in-and-out continues while you sleep and go about your daily business. The depth and rhythm adjust to your level of effort. Just climb those stairs; breathing will take care of itself. Many of us would have died young if breathing required constant attention.

Humans are capable of controlling their breath, though. Cetaceans (whales and dolphins) can, too; must, in fact, and some also use breath control to sing. Other animals can't — or at least don't appear to. Canines in chorus aren't really controlling their breath.

Humans use breath control to generate speech. Humans can make finely controlled exhalation pass over the vocal cords while the length and thickness of the cords is changing to generate different frequencies of sound.

Hemoglobin Dominates Your Red Blood Cells

Hemoglobin is the predominant protein in the red blood cells (RBCs). Specialized for the transport of the blood gases, hemoglobin has the capacity to transport molecular oxygen (attached to the *heme* group) and carbon dioxide (attached to the *globin* portion) simultaneously. In its oxygenated state, it's called *oxyhemoglobin* and is bright red. In the reduced state, it's called *deoxyhemoglobin* and is dark red. Thus the colors of oxygenated arterial and deoxygenated venous blood. (Venous blood isn't blue as it looks through the skin, especially fair skin.)

A typical RBC contains almost nothing but hemoglobin molecules floating in cytoplasm. Hemoglobin makes up about 97 percent of the dry weight of RBCs, and around 35 percent of the total content, including water. The hemoglobin molecules are put together in RBCs as they mature, before the nucleus and other organelles die off. The heme subunits mostly stay together during the four-month life span of the fully differentiated RBC. When the cell dies, the complex is released and broken up in the liver. The iron is salvaged and recycled in new hemoglobin molecules. The rest of the hemoglobin becomes a chemical called *bilirubin,* which is secreted through the bile and into the large intestine, where it gives feces their characteristic yellow-brown color.

Index

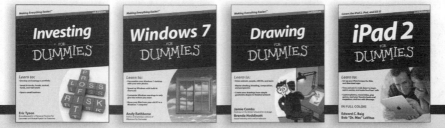

Math & Science

Algebra I
For Dummies,
2nd Edition
978-0-470-55964-2

Biology
For Dummies,
2nd Edition
978-0-470-59875-7

Chemistry
For Dummies,
2nd Edition
978-1-1180-0730-3

Geometry
For Dummies,
2nd Edition
978-0-470-08946-0

Pre-Algebra Essentials
For Dummies
978-0-470-61838-7

Microsoft Office

Excel 2010
For Dummies
978-0-470-48953-6

Office 2010 All-in-One
For Dummies
978-0-470-49748-7

Office 2011 for Mac
For Dummies
978-0-470-87869-9

Word 2010
For Dummies
978-0-470-48772-3

Music

Guitar
For Dummies,
2nd Edition
978-0-7645-9904-0

Clarinet For Dummies
978-0-470-58477-4

iPod & iTunes
For Dummies,
9th Edition
978-1-118-13060-5

Pets

Cats For Dummies,
2nd Edition
978-0-7645-5275-5

Dogs All-in One
For Dummies
978-0470-52978-2

Saltwater Aquariums
For Dummies
978-0-470-06805-2

Religion & Inspiration

The Bible
For Dummies
978-0-7645-5296-0

Catholicism
For Dummies,
2nd Edition
978-1-118-07778-8

Spirituality
For Dummies,
2nd Edition
978-0-470-19142-2

Self-Help & Relationships

Happiness
For Dummies
978-0-470-28171-0

Overcoming Anxiety
For Dummies,
2nd Edition
978-0-470-57441-6

Seniors

Crosswords
For Seniors
For Dummies
978-0-470-49157-7

iPad 2 For Seniors
For Dummies,
3rd Edition
978-1-118-17678-8

Laptops & Tablets
For Seniors
For Dummies,
2nd Edition
978-1-118-09596-6

Smartphones & Tablets

BlackBerry
For Dummies,
5th Edition
978-1-118-10035-6

Droid X2 For Dummies
978-1-118-14864-8

HTC ThunderBolt
For Dummies
978-1-118-07601-9

MOTOROLA XOOM
For Dummies
978-1-118-08835-7

Sports

Basketball
For Dummies,
3rd Edition
978-1-118-07374-2

Football
For Dummies,
2nd Edition
978-1-118-01261-1

Golf For Dummies,
4th Edition
978-0-470-88279-5

Test Prep

ACT For Dummies,
5th Edition
978-1-118-01259-8

ASVAB For Dummies,
3rd Edition
978-0-470-63760-9

The GRE Test
For Dummies,
7th Edition
978-0-470-00919-2

Police Officer Exam
For Dummies
978-0-470-88724-0

Series 7 Exam
For Dummies
978-0-470-09932-2

Web Development

HTML, CSS, & XHTML
For Dummies,
7th Edition
978-0-470-91659-9

Drupal For Dummies,
2nd Edition
978-1-118-08348-2

Windows 7

Windows 7
For Dummies
978-0-470-49743-2

Windows 7
For Dummies,
Book + DVD Bundle
978-0-470-52398-8

Windows 7 All-in-One
For Dummies
978-0-470-48763-1

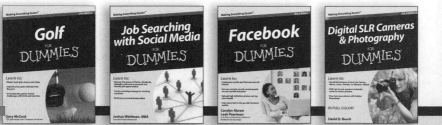

Available wherever books are sold. For more information or to order direct: U.S. customers visit
www.dummies.com or call 1-877-762-2974. U.K. customers visit www.wileyeurope.com or
call (0) 1243 843291. Canadian customers visit www.wiley.ca or call 1-800-567-4797.
Connect with us online at www.facebook.com/fordummies or @fordummies